TABLE OF CONTENTS

LIST OF FIGURES

LIST OF TABLES

PREFACE

The experience of developing a language curriculum for hearing-impaired children has, in many ways, been similar to the experiences seen in some of the fairy tales that have continued to be a source of enjoyment for me.

Central to our story, of course, is a quest—initially for a curriculum outline that would answer every question, solve every problem, and be completely relevant. This unrealistic perspective eventually gave way to the recognition that a curriculum is a process, one in danger of becoming useless if the insights of new information and the dynamics of creativity are missing.

The elusive quest has been a journey full of hopes and frustrations, successes and failures. It has not been a journey traveled alone, however, for there has been the companionship of the fellow authors of this text, the past and present faculty of the Rhode Island School for the Deaf who have shared the risks and results of their daily teaching experience, and the many teachers from past workshops who gave as much as they received. Acknowledgment of these contributions have been made where possible.

Along the way there have been the giants and other strange creatures, frightening at first, but generally harmless and bumbling. In the case of the Rhode Island Department of Education and various grant divisions of the federal government, they have been friendly and helpful.

At the most critical times, when one is not sure of what to do or where to go, there were the mentors and wise ones who advised, directed, or sometimes just encouraged. Among the many, I must recognize the late Clara Hamel without whose insights, hard work, and constant encouragement the journey would not have begun.

The preparation of this manuscript involved many people, but two people in particular deserve special mention; Deborah Topol, whose research and assistance has been invaluable, and Darcy Magratten who designed the book.

Peter M. Blackwell
January 1, 1978

Chapter 1

Introduction and Overview

One of the very disturbing factors encountered when working with hearing-impaired children is their obvious difficulty with "language."

> *"Language is the greatest difficulty the deaf have to overcome in acquiring an education, and they should be given ample time to master it, and the very best teachers to be found should be provided to impart it . . .*
>
> *"One of our most successful instructors of the deaf says: 'A teacher who is imparting idiomatic English may rest assured that she is a good teacher.' She will be able to contrive means that will make the children think of the right things to say and do"* (Annual Report, Rhode Island School for the Deaf, 1896).

As the 1896 document indicates, language is not a new problem, nor is it a problem resulting from a lack of attention. The history of the education of the hearing impaired is replete with names of many creative and dedicated people who have studied, experimented, and attempted to design language development programs. In an attempt to evaluate both the successes and failures of some of these language programs, as well as to contribute some ideas that will address the language problems of hearing-impaired children, several factors need to be carefully identified. The first factor involves the understanding of what is meant by "language."

To define language inadequately surely means that we inadequately define the problem of language acquisition. In this book, language will be viewed as a system which symbolically represents an interrelated set of well-defined relationships. These relationships derive from the cognitive, social, and personal experiences of the child. They are linguistically encoded (or decoded) in the speaker/hearer interaction and may be expressed through oral or manual language or in writing.

Despite the breadth of this definition, language is still more than the sum total of these factors, for the dynamic process of interaction is as important as the product. Teachers must therefore approach language, not as an isolated problem, but as one which functions in joint human interaction. Issues in the acquisition of language, communication, reading, and writing can no longer be lumped together as a general "language" problem. Because language acquisition is not a simple process, solutions to the problems experienced in language learning and teaching cannot be simple either.

It is important to recognize the many teachers who have been successful in the classroom and who have intuitively developed successful language teaching procedures. Many of these approaches, however, are often directly related to the personality or intuitions of these capable and successful teachers and, as such, have not been widely transferable to other classroom situations.

There has been a general trend throughout the history of education of the hearing impaired toward producing a proliferation of oversimplifications with promises for language mastery. Such promises are dependent upon communication systems of various kinds, utilization of media packages, or the introduction of programed curricula. Although some of these activities have met with limited success, it must be clearly stated that the development of language for the hearing-impaired child will never be a simple process. To suggest that it can be so is cruel to the children, parents, and teachers involved.

Apart from the complexities created by a hearing deficit itself, the process of language development for any child is not a simple one to understand. It is only in these last few years that we have gained the barest insight into the language acquisition process of the hearing child, and even more recently into that of the hearing-impaired child. The formulation and proliferation of theories attempting to explain this process have paralleled a rapid change in models of linguistic description. The development of the language curriculum at the Rhode Island School for the Deaf reflects this growth and change in linguistic theories. (*TABLE 1.A*)

Classroom-based language learning in the middle 1960s was geared mainly to the mastery of a list of vocabulary words, which were then built up into simple sentence structures according to a variety of procedures. Even teaching systems that avoided the "structure" of artificial syntax systems seemed to make vocabulary growth the achievement for which teacher and pupil were accountable.

This vocabulary-based language development system resulted from a number of prevailing theories. Firstly, it may have seemed natural that the development of language in young, hearing-impaired children should parallel the development of language in hearing children who, it was believed, merely imitated their parents' words. Secondly, it was probably assumed that vocabulary carries meaning in isolation; that the idea of a noun being the name of a person, place or thing, as well as other similar definitions, adequately described the intrinsic function of words. These words, categorized into "form classes" such as nouns, verbs, adjectives, or other parts of speech, constituted a description of language.

The method of language education then common in programs for the hearing impaired had children associate words with pictures in the early years and study definitions of vocabulary as language became more complex. This approach was based on the assumption that "*. . . . each language contains an arbitrary collection of 'patterns' learned through constant repetition (and 'generalization') and forming a set of 'verbal habits' or 'dispositions'. The belief that language structure and language use can somehow be described in these terms underlies much of the modern study of language and verbal behavior*" (Chomsky, 1964 [in Fodor & Katz, 1965, p. 29]).

Influenced by structural linguistics, this view of language advocated an approach to teaching syntax based on organizing lists of vocabulary in terms of nouns, verbs, adverbs and other parts of speech. These words were then put into appropriate slots following a formula which reflected the various structures of English sentences. An early form of this method, the Barry Five Slate, eventually gave way to the Fitzgerald Key, which is still widely used in programs for deaf children.

A common frustration with such a system is its apparent failure to help students internalize the rules of syntax. The deviant use of language structures by hearing-impaired children is a daily reminder of the inadequacy of this approach and the theory of language from which it grew.

In 1966 the faculty at the Rhode Island School for the Deaf, working with the late Clara Hamel, recognized that a more adequate system of language development was needed. With the encouragement of the principal, Peter M. Blackwell, the faculty began exploring the newly emerging ideas of linguistic theory. Newsome's Structural Grammar in the Classroom (1967), which introduced the concept of "sentence pattern" formula for English sentences and replaced the more cumbersome Fitzgerald Key paradigm, became the basis of the 1971 Rhode Island

LINGUISTIC THEORIES AND RELATED STUDIES IN LANGUAGE DEVELOPMENT	
Prestructuralists *(1870s – 1920s)* Emphasis on philology and word change (the "Neo-Grammarians").	Diary studies (Leopold, 1939–1949; Gregoire, 1937–1947). Informal descriptions (C. Darwin, 1887).
Structuralist/descriptivist *(1950s–1960s)* Emphasis on distribution of phonemes and morphemes in sentences. Attempts in classifying parts of speech using a taxonomic method (Harris, 1951).	Emphasis on the acquisition of phonemes, morphemes and surface structure frames (Braine, 1963; Brown, Fraser, & Bellugi, 1964).
Transformational Grammar *(1960s – present)* Emphasis on syntactic relationships within and between sentences based on a system of underlying rules (Chomsky, 1965).	Emphasis on the acquisition of phrase structure rules and transformational rules (Menyuk, 1969; McNeill, 1966; Brown & Hanlon, 1970).
Semantically-based grammars; case grammars *(1970s)* Emphasis on the relationship between language structures and meaning (Fillmore, 1968; Chafe, 1970).	Emphasis on discovering how a child conveys meaning with word relationships and on the acquisition of semantic features (Bloom, 1970; E. Clark, 1973).
Functionally-based grammars *(1970s)* Emphasis on the context in which language is used and its function in social interaction.	Emphasis on how children use language in social contexts (Nelson, 1973; Bruner, 1975).

TABLE 1.A Linguistic theories and related studies in language development

Curriculum. The idea of predictable separate sentence structures was certainly more manageable for teachers and children than the Key headings but did not seem to make much difference in the overall mastery of syntax.

Newsome's perspectives emphasized the application of structural linguistics to the classroom, a reasonable beginning as the structuralists were among the few linguists writing anything for the classroom at that time. These ideas were also seen in the early Roberts' English series (1966) and later in the Apple Tree program (1973) written especially for hearing-impaired students. But although these systems of building sentences were simple, they still assumed that vocabulary in isolation was the appropriate starting place. Also the level of syntax did not go beyond the simple sentence and it emphasized "straight language" rather than complex language.

It was around this time that the field of linguistics began to rapidly expand, mainly as a result of interest in the transformational-generative grammar of Noam Chomsky. The concept of transformational-generative grammar raised several critical questions relevant to a language development curriculum. However, Chomsky's ideas were considered extremely radical at the time and the early Rhode Island School for the Deaf's curricula reflected a syncretizing of transformational grammar perspectives with some "security blankets" of structuralism, such as vocabulary lists and an overriding interest in the form of sentences.

Firstly, Chomsky influenced the thinking of students of child language acquisition, such as Paula Menyuk (who in turn questioned the importance of isolated vocabulary), by pointing out that the meaning and part of speech assigned to a word is determined by its relationship to other vocabulary in a sentence.

"In a sentence the Subject is the Noun Phrase of the sentence, Object is the Noun Phrase of the Verb Phrase and the Predicate is the Verb Phrase of the sentence. Thus the class Noun and Verb are defined by functions in sentences.

"To understand and generate sentences the child must observe the functional relationships in a sentence, then define types of classifications, and then observe selectional constraints on the combinations of these classes (Menyuk, 1969, p. 23).

Secondly, Chomsky introduced the concept of two levels of sentence functioning; that which is actually spoken or heard at the surface level, called surface structure, and the underlying level which reflects the actual meaning of the sentence, the deep structure. Between these two levels operate predictable transformational rules, which in essence "transform" meaning into actual utterances.

What is important in language functioning is that students learn to recognize the deep structure of sentences, particularly as sentences increase in complexity. This process involves understanding the relationship between deep and surface structures and the transformations that relate the two. Studies by Quigley et al. (1976), however, show that hearing-impaired students do not seem to use this deep structure widely and are so dependent upon surface structure functioning that they have great difficulty handling language containing transformations of any complexity.

By the time the staff of the Rhode Island School for the Deaf was ready for a program based on the syntactic perspectives of Chomsky's Syntactic Structures (1957), the field of linguistics itself had moved on. It was now seriously considering the issues of semantics, cognition, social relationships, neurophysiology, semiotics and a host of other factors for which no neat, manageable grammars have been written. New insights encouraged richer and more sophisticated studies of child language acquisition by psychologists and linguists, which in turn encouraged the application of further insights to the teaching of language at the Rhode Island School for the Deaf.

Although there have been significant changes in the curriculum, motivated by both the general growth in knowledge of language development in children and by the information gathered from experience in the classrooms, we have only scratched the surface of a language development curriculum. There is no pretense here to present a simple and final package of what a teacher should do.

Fortunately, it is not only the proliferation of knowledge that necessitates the inclusion of the foregoing factors in the curriculum. The students themselves have indicated, in their expanding mastery of language, the many issues apart from syntax that must be considered in a complete language development curriculum.

One finds here the work of many people who have contributed to the development of this curriculum through their research, dialogue, teaching, and learning. The ideas presented must be kept alive by being constantly open to this process.

ACKNOWLEDGMENTS

QUOTES

Page 4 From *Sentences Children Use* by Paula Menyuk, 1969. Copyright © 1969 by M.I.T. Press. Reprinted by permission of the publisher.

Chapter 2

Cognitive and Linguistic Development

The development of a student's cognitive ability is one goal common to most educational programs. In educational programs for the hearing impaired, the development of language is always another goal. When developing a curriculum it seems helpful to first investigate theories of cognitive and linguistic development or, perhaps more importantly, the areas where they intersect to see what theoretical studies these areas have to offer. Some aspects of cognitive and linguistic development will be presented here as a basis for discussing an overall approach to curriculum design and language education.

The wealth of terminology presented here represents explorations in many areas, but due to space limitations only the barest skeleton of a very full-bodied theory is offered. Therefore, the theories and terms included are those we find most useful. In a rapidly changing field, these theories and our relationship to these theories are also likely to change rapidly.

Cognitive Studies

Piaget

Some of the most extensive studies in child development come from Jean Piaget. Although many of his publications date back to the 1920s, it is only recently that educators have been influenced by the work of the famous Swiss psychologist. According to Piaget's model of cognitive development, a child in a preschool program (2 to 6 years old) is considered to be in the **preoperational stage** of cognitive development. At 5 or 6 years of age, the child enters the stage of **concrete operations** and then eventually moves into the stage of **formal operations** somewhere between 10 and 14 years of age. *(TABLE 2.B)*

The first two years of life are defined by Piaget as the period of **sensorimotor** intelligence. During this period the child goes through a process of finding an equilibrium between adapting to the environment–**accommodation** in Piagetian terms–and acting upon the environment–**assimilation.**

Piaget's Stages of Intellectual Development	
ONE	The Sensorimotor Stage (*0 to 18 months*)
TWO	The Preoperational Stage (*18 months to age 7*)
THREE	Concrete Operations (*7 to 12 years*)
FOUR	Formal Operations (*12 years and onward*)

Table 2.B Piaget's stages of intellectual development

The pattern of behavior that grows from this interaction between accommodation and assimilation is described as a **schema**, which is the child's representation of experience. The schema makes it possible for the child to reproduce a certain action at will. Throughout the developmental process, schemas become integrated by undergoing a process of accommodation and assimilation with each other. During the preoperational stage, this process of integration expands as the child establishes relationships between experience and action. *(FIGURE 2.1)*

Pooh Invents a New Game: Accommodation/Assimilation

"One day, when Pooh was walking towards this bridge he was trying to make up a piece of poetry about fir-cones, because there they were lying about on each side of him, and he felt singy. So, he picked a fir-cone up, and looked at it . . . He had just come to the bridge; and not looking where he was going, he tripped over something and the fir-cone jerked out of his paw into the river.
" 'Bother', said Pooh, as it floated under the bridge and he went back to get another fir-cone which had a rhyme to it. But then he thought that he would just look at the river instead, because it was a peaceful sort of day, so he lay down and looked at it, and it slipped slowly away beneath him . . . . . and suddenly, there was his fir-cone slipping away too. 'That's funny', said Pooh. 'I dropped it on the other side', said Pooh, 'and it came out on this side! I wonder if it would do it again?' "

Pooh is accommodating in a number of ways here. First, having picked up the fir-cone, he trips and the fir-cone falls into the river. He does not intend this to happen and he goes to get another fir-cone. He coincidentally lies down and looks at the river from the other side of the bridge and notices that his fir-cone has floated under the bridge.

At this point Pooh reasons that this process, which initially happened by accident, might be repeated deliberately.

"It did. It kept on doing it. Then he dropped two in at once, and leant over the bridge to see which of them would come out first, and one of them did; but as they were both the same size, he didn't know if it was the one he wanted to win, or the other one."

Here Pooh assimilates the action of dropping the fir-cone in the river and modifies his new mastery by dropping in two fir-cones. However, he accommodates to this new experience because he cannot tell the difference between the fir-cones.

"So the next time he dropped one big one and one little one, and the big one came out first, which was, what he said it would do, and the little one came out last which was what he said it would do, so he won twice . . . ."

FIGURE 2.1 The learning process that grows from accommodation and assimilation is clearly seen in A. A. Milne's House at Pooh Corner, *where "Pooh Invents a New Game and Everyone Joins In."*

Piaget (1926) notes, though, that the child does not distinguish between feelings and external reality at this time and therefore, in accommodation to perceptual experience, is likely to say that the clouds move because we move, or the stars, like us, have to go to bed. In the attempt to assimilate reality, the child is unable to separate goals from the means of achieving them, and when forced to change activities because he is unable to manipulate reality, the child does so by intuitive or external regulation rather than by symbolic or internal operations.

What the child has not developed during this period is the concept of **reversibility.** For example, the very young child cannot grasp the idea that if one changes the shape of a ball of clay, it can readily be restored to its original shape. In order to understand the relationships involved in restoring the clay to its original shape, the child would have to understand the relationship between dimensions or attributes of the clay. This would be **conservation,** a key Piagetian term. In other words, a child cannot carry out the operation of reversibility on the clay because he does not understand the relationships between the salient attributes and cannot conserve them in an internalized, symbolic form. Reversibility, then, is a critical aspect of conservation, which is gradually mastered throughout the stage of concrete operations.

COGNITIVE STUDIES AND THE EDUCATION OF THE HEARING IMPAIRED

In certain situations, teachers may be asking pupils to utilize material appropriate for most children at a given age but unsuitable for others who have not mastered conservation in that area. According to psychologist Mireille de Meuron and psychiatrist Edgar H. Auerswald, *"School curricula do not make provisions for cognitive deficits, they help perpetuate the dyssocial behavior bred by these deficits"* (Roche, 1967, p. 17). It was noted in their study of 57 chronically misbehaving children from low-income families that *"typically a child enters the third cognitive stage, characterized by the development of logical thinking, at seven or eight, but none of these problem children had arrived at this stage 'on time.' Most were ten or eleven years old when this characteristic appeared"* (Roche, 1967, p. 17).

At this stage, the process of integrating information and the educational process of mastering material involve the conflict between perceptual and symbolic representation. Influenced mainly by perceptual information, the preoperational child perceives that a beaker of water poured into a taller, thinner beaker increases in volume because its height increases. The child eventually learns to modify the perceptual experience through symbolic representation in an appropriate learning environment. The hearing-impaired child at this age often has not developed a mature enough system of symbolic representation to assimilate the environment and therefore accommodates to the perceptual experience.

The preceding example may provide some understanding of the findings of Hans Furth (1966), who reported that deaf children were about one year and seven months delayed in developing the processes of conservation of weight and they also exhibited a similar lag in most other Piagetian tasks. Although Sinclair-de Zwart (1969) does not feel that this lag is significant, it should be remembered that most tests using Piagetian tasks have concentrated on the stage of concrete operations. It would not be surprising to find that the delay in hearing-impaired children entering the stage of formal operations is significant, particularly as it is this stage that requires sophistication in symbolic representation.

After also noticing the cognitive delay in deaf children, Oléron (1957) observed that Piaget's theory does not sufficiently emphasize the role of language in the development of cognition. Piaget divides the functioning of children's language into two developmental stages. First, there is **egocentric speech** emerging out of noncommunicative thought. Included in this category would be language play, where the child repeats for pleasure of talking (a type of accommodation), and monologue and dual monologue, which in turn are types of experimentation not defined earlier.

The second stage in the development of speech, according to Piaget, is **socialized speech.** This includes speech that contains adapted information, criticism, commands, requests or threats, questions and answers, all of which are language functions indicating assimilation. However, Piaget does not specifically emphasize the importance of language as a major influence on cognitive organization.

Vygotsky

The influential Russian psychologist Vygotsky, on the other hand, not only specifically notes the influence of language on cognitive development, but reverses the order of Piaget's stages of speech development. Vygotsky (1934) notes that social speech develops first and then, when the child's inner psychic functioning begins, egocentric speech appears. This "thinking aloud" is then internalized as inner thought or **inner language.**

Whereas Piaget emphasizes sensorimotor development as the foundation for symbolization, Vygotsky says that thought development is determined by language and the sociocultural experiences of the child. For Vygotsky, inner language is a late development and is the result of realistic thought and its corollary, thinking in concepts. This kind of cognitive development enables the individual to achieve a degree of autonomy from reality and, perhaps, find in imagination the satisfaction of needs frustrated in life.

The thinking of Vygotsky should encourage reevaluation of the current traditional methods of teaching language through basically unorganized vocabulary without due emphasis on concept formation. The emphasis on language through concept development and the notion that actions will be encouraged and modified by language are two important ideas drawn from Vygotsky's work that are of value in curriculum development.

Bruner

A third cognitive psychologist whose work is of great interest and value to teachers is Jerome Bruner, who has expressed some reservations about Vygotsky's claims concerning language influencing actions. According to Bruner, *"if one is using symbolic representation to guide action, the success of the effort will depend upon the extent to which the sphere of experience or action has been prepared to bring it into some conformance with the requirements of language"* (Bruner et al., 1966, p. 55). As an alternative, Bruner presents a model that accounts for the important factors covered in the approaches of Piaget and Vygotsky and one that may provide a more useful perspective for shaping an educational program for hearing-impaired children.

Bruner notes three systems, each unique and somewhat parallel, by which we represent the experience of the world and the impact of culture on shaping growth. **Enactive processes** involve representation by action and experimentation similar to processes in Piaget's sensorimotor stage. **Iconic representation** is established through perceptual imagery, such as pictures or diagrams. The third system, **symbolic representation,** is different from Piaget's mental imagery and involves mainly language. *(FIGURE 2.2)*

But most important is Bruner's emphasis on language as a means of organizing experience. *"I would argue that language itself is not what is 'imposed' on experience, as already suggested in my rejection of Vygotsky's idea that language is internalized and becomes inner speech which is tantamount to thought. Rather, language comes from the same basic root out of which symbolically organized experience grows . . . It is by the interaction of language and the barely symbolically organized experience of the child of two or three that language gradually finds its way into the realm of experience"* (Bruner et al., 1966, p. 43).

COGNITION AND CURRICULUM DESIGN

Bruner's work emphasizes the relationship of language and cognition in the growing child. Herbert Clark (1973), in discussing how a child acquires the language to express concepts of space and time, examines this relationship.

". . . the child acquires English expression for space and time by learning how to apply these expressions to the a priori knowledge he has about space and time. This a priori knowledge is separate from language itself and is not so mysterious. The knowledge, it will be argued, is simply what the child knows about space given that he lives on this planet, has a particular perceptual apparatus, and moves around in a characteristic manner. The exact form of this knowledge, then, is dependent on man's biological endowment—that he has two eyes, ears, etc . . . , that he stands upright, and so on—and in this sense it is innate. For the present, however, it is more constructive to consider the present paper within a cognitive framework. The thesis is simply that the child knows much about space and time before he learns the English terms for space and time, and his acquisition of these terms is built onto his prior cognitive development" (p. 28).

THREE SYSTEMS OF REPRESENTATION IN THE CLASSROOM

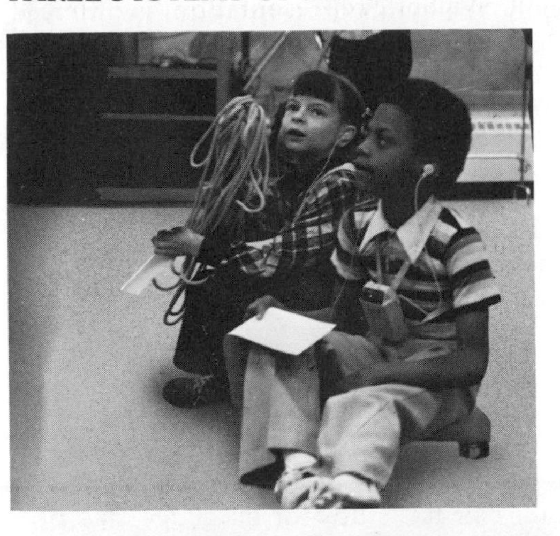

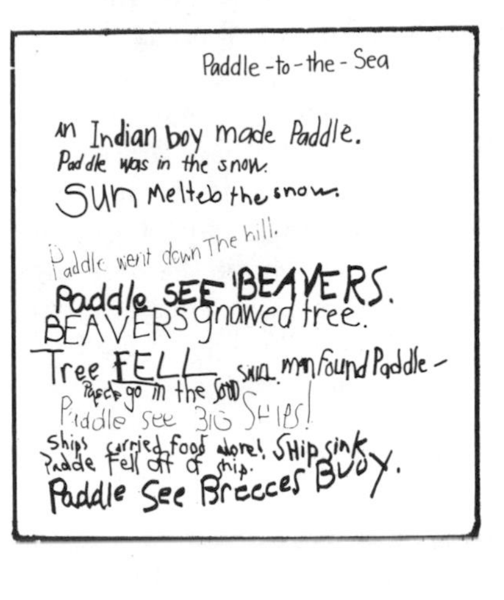
Paddle-to-the-Sea
An Indian boy made Paddle.
Paddle was in the snow.
SUN Melteb the snow.
Paddle went down The hill.
Paddle SEE BEAVERS.
BEAVERS gnawed tree.
Tree FELL
Paddle see BIG SHIPS!
Ships carried food alone! SHIP sink.
Paddle Fell off of ship.
Paddle See Breeces BUOY.

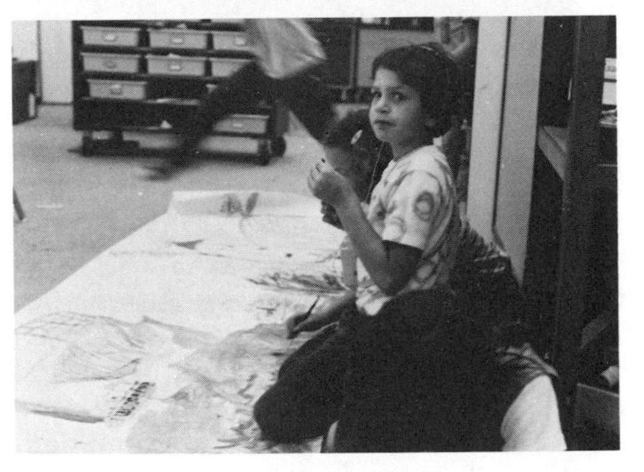

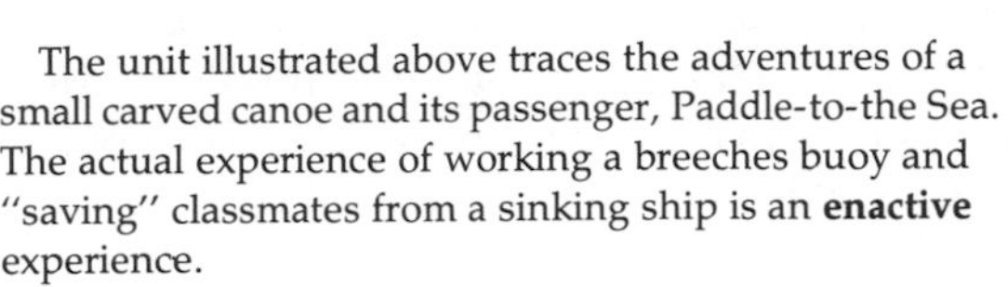

The unit illustrated above traces the adventures of a small carved canoe and its passenger, Paddle-to-the Sea. The actual experience of working a breeches buoy and "saving" classmates from a sinking ship is an **enactive** experience.

Each of the children's drawings which recreate the experience are **iconic** representations, since there is a one-to-one correspondence between the drawing (or signifier) and the experience itself (the signified).

The third mode of representation used in this unit is the **symbolic.** In this mode the enactive or iconic modes are made symbolic by their representation in language.

FIGURE 2.2 Three systems of representation in the classroom.

Language plays some kind of integrating role, shifting the enactive and iconic cognitive experiences, which are largely perceptually based, to a linguistically based representation through which more appropriate categorization and generalization can occur.

The principle for curriculum design seems clear; experiences must not only be represented enactively and iconically in the classroom, but must be moved to the symbolic, that is linguistic, level of representation. Should there be an imbalance in this relationship, deficits may occur in the cognitive and/or linguistic development of the child.

For example, it is not unusual for hearing-impaired children to be exposed, particularly in the early years, to a curriculum based on a variety of experiences. The teaching process remains largely enactive and iconic. However, particularly if the language chosen for classroom use is only vocabulary matched with pictures, the vocabulary words intended as symbolic representations of experience become instead only iconic representations.

Certainly Bruner's theory would have one question the efficiency of a system or curriculum that did not have an appropriate balance between symbolic representation (language input) and other forms of representing experience. There is, in fact, a serious question as to whether real learning takes place in this kind of setting, for the paucity of language does not adequately organize the experiences so that the child may internalize them. It is the reconsideration of the relationship between cognition and language that has led to the reevaluation of the hearing-impaired child's learning experience and curricula, which have been the basis of education of the hearing impaired for many years.

COGNITIVE STYLES

The imbalance of cognitive and linguistic experiences may help to explain the observation made by Dr. Toby Silverman (1968) that hearing-impaired people seem to have a functionally oriented cognitive style. Silverman defines three categories of cognitive style. The first is the primitive or "folk society" where existence in an agrarian-based economy is perceptually oriented. Color, size and shape are important, and behavior is motivated by differences in these attributes.

On the other hand, the technological society, whose cognitive organization is based on similarities realized in categories, has a complex culture with a process of ordering and labeling called superordination. Superordinates have no direct representation. There is no one thing that can be pointed at to define food, furniture, or justice. These abstractions help in ordering the complex technical world.

There is also an intermediate cognitive style utilizing a functional type of thinking. Silverman believes that the hearing impaired are functionally oriented in that they *"neither use predominately perceptual features such as color, size, or shape, nor do they recognize superordinate categories"* (Silverman, 1968, unpublished).

If the hearing-impaired student is to become a successful member of technological society, then that student will have to develop the appropriate cognitive style. And, it is only the symbolic representation of language that will enable the child to organize objects and events and modify perceptual representations in order to reach this goal.

Linguistics and Language Acquisition

SOME WAYS OF TALKING ABOUT LANGUAGE

The tremendous interest during the last two decades in the study of language has produced a wealth of theories about the acquisition and structure of language, a large family of subfields (psycholinguistics, sociolinguistics, neurolinguistics, etc.) and a predictable proliferation of technical terminology. The language development approach presented here draws on many of these theories and subfields and tries to extract from them what is valuable for education of the hearing impaired. As a result, terminology has been mixed from diverse areas within linguistics, some definitions have been loosened, and some theories bent; hopefully no term, definition, or theory has been distorted beyond its reasonable scope while blending them to construct the linguistic basis for a language development program.

The aspects of modern linguistics presented here do not represent a complete survey of modern linguistic science. Rather, only those aspects of modern linguistics that were found useful in developing and discussing a language curriculum for language-delayed and language-disordered students are presented. Also presented are those aspects of linguistics that teachers find useful, those that provide tools for the assessment of language ability, and those aspects that students themselves make use of in their language acquisition.

THEORIES OF GRAMMAR

"The heart of human language capability is creativity in expressing and understanding meanings . . . 'appropriate to new and ever changing situations.' It can be explained only if what we know in common with other members of our language community is a finite set of rules. These rules express the relationships that hold between meaning and sound in our particular language, and they channel our creativity within the limits of intelligibility and appropriateness for our speech community.

"A description of such a set of rules is called grammar. Like all descriptions of natural phenomena, grammars are subject to continuous revision and correction. In the range of phenomena they explain, the most powerful grammars of adult English are generative transformational grammars first written by a group of linguists centering around Noam Chomsky" (Cazden, 1972, p. 6–7).

Transformational-generative theory is the basis of the language development approach, although it must be recognized that this basic theory has gone through many stages and changes. The basic sentence pattern approach in the 1971 Rhode Island School Curriculum finds its roots in the early transformational grammars of Harris (1964) and Chomsky (1957), while current approaches to complex sentences grow out of later work in transformational grammars (Rosenbaum, 1967; Ross, 1967). Much of our thinking about semantics has been influenced by generative semantics (Ross, 1970; 1975), the case grammar proposals of Fillmore (1968), and a semiotic approach inspired by Roman Jakobson (1968).

Still at the root of the approach is the concept of a **grammar** as a system of rules that organize linguistic representations. When discussing language in this book, both that underlying system–the grammar–and the actual linguistic representations that the grammar allows one to produce and understand are implied in its definition. Linguistic representations include speech, signs, symbols, print and other ways of organizing and representing meaning. The grammar is called **generative** because it is infinitely productive; it allows for the understanding and production of an unlimited range of meanings through a rule-governed system. A **transformational grammar,** then, is a model of the system of mental rules that allow people to generate and comprehend linguistic representations. It is a system for producing and understanding sentences.

Chomsky

That a generative grammar is many things, from a somewhat mechanistic system of generating strings of language to an abstract series of mental rules, can be seen in this succession of quotes from the originator of the generative grammar concept:

"The grammar of a Language will thus be a device that generates all of the grammatical sequences of that Language and none of the ungrammatical ones" (Chomsky, 1957, p. 13).

"A grammar, in the traditional view, is an account of competence. It describes and attempts to account for the ability of the speaker to understand an arbitrary sentence of his language and to produce an appropriate sentence on a given occasion . . . . A generative grammar is a system of rules that relates signals to semantic interpretations of these signals" (Chomsky, 1966, p. 10).

". . . . by a generative grammar I mean simply a system of rules that in some explicit and well defined way assigns structural descriptions to sentences. Obviously, every speaker of a language has mastered and internalized a generative grammar that expressed his knowledge of his language . . . . Any interesting generative grammar will be dealing, for the most part, with mental processes that are far beyond the level of actual or even potential consciousness; . . . thus a generative grammar attempts to specify what a speaker actually knows" (Chomsky, 1965, p. 8).

This broad conception of a generative grammar is the basis for the Rhode Island School for the Deaf Language Development Curriculum, and the development of a generative grammar in each student is the goal of that curriculum. As Chomsky (1966) notes, *"A linguistic grammar aims to discover and exhibit the mechanisms that make this achievement (language) possible . . . . If it is a pedagogic grammar, it attempts to provide the student with this ability"* (p. 10).

GENERATIVE GRAMMAR

In brief, a generative grammar is made up of interrelated components. The two of most concern here are the syntactic and semantic components. **Syntax** generally refers to the structure of sentences, their word order, and the changes that take place in word order or sentence structure as sentences vary in meaning, style, or function.

Sentences are the basic unit of a transformational-generative grammar (T-G) and are a useful organizing unit for curriculum design as well. Sentences have a **deep structure** and a **surface structure.** The surface structure is the actual form of the sentence produced or the sentence to be understood. This surface form may be produced and/or comprehended through speech, sign, or, in the case of the printed code, reading or writing. The deep structure is the underlying representation of the sentence and is closely related to its meaning. The **semantic component** of the grammar is that which interprets and generates the underlying meaning relationships in the deep structure.

The operations that relate deep and surface structures are **transformations.** When linguists refer to rules of grammar they are referring either to the rules for putting together meanings in the deep structure (the phrase structure rules) or rules for relating deep structure to surface structure representations (transformations). Deep structure, thus, begins to take on the appearance of semantic representation of the sentence, for the grammatical relationships that are expressed in deep structure are as important to the meaning of a sentence as the words (the **lexical items**) themselves.

Two other aspects of a generative grammar are the **phonological** and the **morphological components.** Morphology generally refers to processes that can occur at the word level; for example, the addition of *-ly* to adverbs or past tense endings to verbs. Morphological processes are related to syntax, as in the case of changing adjectives into adverbs, and are important in the expression of semantic relationships, as in the past tense ending.

Morphological processes are often reflected in changes in the sounds of words, such as the addition of plural *-s*. These changes are reflected in the phonology, the sound system of a language. And, when considering the interrelatedness of these components of a generative language system–the semantic as expressed in the syntactic, morphological, and phonological processes of linguistic representation–it is apparent that speech problems are not simply circumscribed phonological problems independent of overall linguistic representation, language structure and function.

Considerations of the form of a generative grammar lead to the two important concepts in the theory of transformational-generative grammar. They are **competence** and **performance,** and these lead inevitably to the distinction between speech and language. According to Chomsky (1965), *"we thus make a fundamental distinction between competence (the speaker/hearer's knowledge of his language) and performance, the actual use of language in concrete situations"* (p. 4).

The generative grammar purports to be a description of the ideal speaker/hearer's competence. While the two are not the same, the surface structure is a closer representation of the speaker's performance while the deep structure is more a description of competence. The use of transformations relating deep to surface structure is also part of the native speaker's competence, as well as the ability of the speaker to understand sentences in terms of their underlying meanings and relationships. An even more complex aspect of linguistic competence is the ability of the native speaker/hearer to integrate and use the phonological, morphological, syntactic and semantic components in the expressive and receptive performances of linguistic acts.

Seen in this light, speech is not the same as language. Speech is the actual phonetic expression, and language is the total system behind that production. While the phonological component is clearly related to speech, it is only part of the overall system of language with its own deep and surface aspects.

Recent work of Bellugi and Klima (1975) and Stokoe (1975) indicates that American Sign Language is a developed language in the fullest sense of the word. While the relationships between competence and performance and deep and surface structures in manual languages have not been fully explicated, one would expect that these theoretical constructs apply in this area as well as to oral languages.

Oral languages of the world vary greatly in surface forms, while in their underlying systematicity there is much less variation. This commonality in language organization leads not only to the search for language universals, but to language development programs that seek to develop in the child an organized system of language regardless of the particular language, dialect, or mode.

LANGUAGE ACQUISITION

With all of the above descriptions and models of language, there remains the problem of trying to apply grammars formulated for adult language to the language of children. Since the ultimate goal of the child's language development is an adult grammar, the two cannot be formulated independently. However, to date, a grammar that is suitable for both adult and child language has not been conceived.

In the study of child language several stages of development are apparent. Early studies, predating the development of syntactic theories, concentrated mainly on describing the acquisition of vocabulary since that was what language was thought to be (McCarthy, 1954). In addition there were a number of so-called "diary" studies which were descriptions, usually by parents, of the grammatical development of a child's productive language over a period of several years (i.e., Leopold, 1949; Gregoire, 1937; Darwin, 1877 [in Bar Adon & Leopold, 1971]).

Charles Darwin's "Biographical Sketch of an Infant" exemplifies this type of study.

"At exactly the age of a year, he made the great step of inventing a word for food, namely, 'mum,' but what led him to it I did not discover. And now instead of beginning to cry when he was hungry, he used this word in a demonstrative manner or as a verb, implying 'give me food.' But he also used 'mum' as a substantive of wide signification; thus he called sugar 'shu-mum,' and a little later after he had learned the word 'black,' he called liquorice 'black-shu-mum'—black-sugar-food, . . .

Finally, the wants of an infant are at first made intelligible by instinctive cries, which after a time are modified in part unconsciously, and in part, as I believe, voluntarily as a means of communication—by the gestures as well as several words and short sentences" (Darwin, 1877 [in Bar-Adon & Leopold, 1971, p. 26]).

As linguists became more sophisticated about the nature of language, studies of child language changed accordingly. During the 1960s much of the research concentrated on specific areas of acquisition, such as question formation (Brown, 1968), morphological inflections (Berko, 1958; Cazden, 1968), and the development of syntax (Menyuk, 1964, 1969, 1971; Braine, 1963, 1971; McNeill, 1970).

During this period of growth in the field, several terms were widely used in the characterization of child language. **Holophrastic** was, and still is, used to convey the belief that the child's first single words often function as a complete statement or sentence. That is, children do not simply name, but comment on objects or events, give commands, reject commands, or express possession. One might assume that the child has a complete idea in mind but does not have the linguistic structure available to express it. Holophrastic speech is interpreted in many different ways, however, depending on whether one assumes that the child has a full sentence in mind (McNeill, 1970) or interprets one-word utterances more narrowly (Bloom, 1973).

"In summary, single-word utterances are not sentences. Children in the first half of the second year do not use phrases and sentences—they say only one word at a time. When single-word utterances are successive, within the bounds of a single speech event, there is some evidence to indicate that the child is aware of relational aspects of experience. But children do not use syntax—utterances are largely unpredictable relative to one another—and there is no evidence from their linguistic performance that children 'know' the semantic-syntactic structure of the language that they hear . . . .

"It appears then that children say only one word at a time primarily because they do not yet know the linguistic code. Although no doubt cognizant of certain relations in experience, they are unable to code such experience linguistically" (Bloom, 1973, p. 61–63).

From our point of view it is important to consider how the utterances of a hearing-impaired child at a one-word stage compare to those of a hearing child. Since the hearing-impaired child arrives at this stage later (chronologically) and remains at this level for a longer period, one questions what he is expressing with his word. Is he naming or commenting, for instance? If he is delayed in acquiring syntax, is it more likely that he is expressing an idea with his one word?

Early child language is also sometimes characterized as **telegraphic.** This term stems from the resemblance between the child's language when he first attempts sentences and the language of a telegram in which redundant or nonessential words which make the message more expensive are eliminated. The child at this stage, because of a constraint on length or sentence complexity, uses sentences made up largely of nouns and verbs with a few adjectives and adverbs (i.e., content words). What is missing are the less essential **function words** such as determiners, prepositions, conjunctions and verbal auxiliaries. Function words are defined aptly by Brown (1973) as words that do not make reference but rather mark grammatical structures, carry subtle modulatory meanings, and do not readily admit new members. The language of hearing-impaired children far older than the children in many studies of early language acquisition is often described as telegraphic.

Roger Brown

Many contributions to the study of child language have come from Roger Brown, whose work has spanned the entire period from the late 1950s to the present. Most of the early approaches to the study of child language are described and evaluated in detail in his book A First Language (1973).

One of his contributions to the methodology of language sampling was the use of the **MLU (mean length of utterance)** as a measure of language development. Since age is not a good basis for comparing children's language because rates of development vary so greatly, many regular aspects of development are revealed when children are compared by this measure. The MLU is based on the smallest meaningful element (morpheme) rather than words and is defined as the average length of the child's utterances in morphemes. Brown (1973) gives precise rules for the calculation of MLU. The MLU is a good index of grammatical development because

The Order of Acquisition of 14 Grammatical Morphemes in Three Children

MLU	Age	Adam		Sarah		Eve
1.75	I(2;3)		I(2;3)		1(1;6)	
2.25	II(2;6)	Present progressive *in* *on*, plural	II(2;10)	Plural *in, on*	II(1;9)	
				Present progressive past irregular Possessive		Present progressive, *on*
2.75	III(2;11)		III(3;1)		III(1;11)	*in*
		Uncontractible copula, past irregular		Uncontractible copula Articles		
						Plural, possessive
3.50	IV(3;2)		IV(3;8)		IV(2;2)	Past regular
		Articles Third person irregular possessive		Third person regular		
4:00	V(3;6)	Third person regular Past regular Uncontractible auxiliary Contractible copula Contractible auxiliary	V(4;0)	Past regular Uncontractible auxiliary Contractible copula Third person irregular Contractible copula	V(2;3)	Uncontractible copula Past irregular Articles Third person regular Third person irregular Uncontractible auxiliary Contractible copula Contractible auxiliary

Source: Roger Brown, *A First Language,* 1973, p. 271.

TABLE 2.C The order of acquisition of 14 grammatical morphemes in three children

new knowledge expressed in the surface form of a sentence always increases length. Therefore, two children matched for MLU are more likely to be on the same level of complexity than two children of the same chronological age.

This measure provides a background for using stages to describe a child's language. Brown (1973) has proposed Stage I for the period beginning with the first multiword utterances and continuing until MLU reaches 2.0. The subsequent stages increase by increments of 0.5.

TABLE 2.C illustrates the order of acquisition of grammatical morphemes through Stage V, or an MLU of 4.00. That is, hearing children at Stage V will usually express tense, plurality, possession, the verb *to be,* etc.

A question to consider at this point is, since the hearing-impaired child has usually not acquired these grammatical morphemes by Stage V, how this affects his further development of language.

Proceeding hand-in-hand with the data-collecting studies and description of that data were the theories of how the child learns language. Two ideas from the field of psychology, imitation and reinforcement, had considerable impact on the thinking in this area. The theories stated that children simply imitate what they hear adults say, and the reinforcement they receive from adult speakers for their correct utterances teaches them appropriate usage.

Chomsky (1964 [in Fodor & Katz, 1965]), in his review of Skinner's Verbal Behavior, discusses these possibilities as explanation of the child's acquisition of language.

"*. . . it seems quite beyond question that children acquire a good deal of verbal and nonverbal behavior by casual observation and imitation of adults and other children. It is simply not true that children can learn language only through 'meticulous care' on the part of adults who shape their verbal repertoire through careful differential reinforcement . . . As far as acquisition of language is concerned, it seems clear that reinforcement, casual observation and natural inquisitiveness (coupled with a strong tendency to imitate) are important factors as is the remarkable capacity of the child to generalize, hypothesize and 'process information' in a variety of very special and apparently highly complex ways which we cannot yet describe or begin to understand and which may be largely innate, or may develop through some sort of learning or through maturation of the nervous system . . . . The fact that all normal children acquire essentially comparable grammars of great complexity with remarkable rapidity suggests that human beings are somehow specially designed to do this, with data-handling or 'hypothesis-formulating' ability of unknown character and complexity*" (p. 562–563).

There is by now fairly strong evidence that imitation and reinforcement as an explanation for language development is inadequate (Brown & Hanlon, 1970). The experimental evidence offered by the studies of Lenneberg (1962); Bloom et al. (1974); Brown, Cazden, and Bellugi (1969); and Nelson (1973) for instance, shows clearly that a child would be unable to formulate a grammar based on what they describe as the incomplete and fragmented data of the adult language he hears.

Expansions of Child Speech Produced By Mothers

Child	Mother
Baby highchair	Baby is in the highchair.
Mommy eggnog	Mommy had her eggnog.
Eve lunch	Eve is having lunch.
Mommy sandwich	Mommy'll have a sandwich.
Sat well	He sat on the wall.
Throw Daddy	Throw it to Daddy.
Pick glove	Pick the glove up.

Source: Roger Brown, *A First Language,* 1973, p. 105.

TABLE 2.D Expansions of child speech produced by mothers

Another aspect of child/parent interaction considered as a possible means by which the child learns language is expansion and modeling. That is, adults interpret a child's sentence by utilizing context and supplying the missing elements, such as function words, to build the utterance into a complete sentence. (*TABLE 2.D.*) Although it seems reasonable that this kind of feedback would serve as good training for the child, Cazden (1965), for one, did not find any evidence that expansions were effective in helping the child toward more complete utterances.

One of the other early characterizations of child language coming from this period was the pivot-open grammar of Martin Braine (1963). A pivot grammar utilizes just two word classes, pivot and open, and the rules generate only two-word sentences. Neither telegraphic nor pivot characterizations interpret from the data, nor do they try to describe what the child means by his utterances.

These early approaches are no longer thought to be descriptive enough or accurate enough characterizations of child language (Bloom, 1970; Brown, 1973; Bowerman, 1973). The addition of contextual information was an important contribution of Bloom's 1970 and 1973 studies. She supplied complete records of the context of each utterance and was therefore able to hypothesize about what meaning was intended. Dale (1976) describes Bloom's methodology:

". . . Bloom (1970) kept very complete records of the context of each utterance and was able in many cases to formulate a more precise hypothesis about the meaning intended. One of the children she studied, Kathryn, provided a particularly striking example of the value of context. Kathryn said mommy sock *twice in one day, once when she picked up her mother's sock and again when her mother put Kathryn's own sock on her. Clearly the relationship between* mommy *and* sock *differs in these two utterances; in the first,* mommy *is a possessive modifier of sock, whereas in the second,* mommy *is the agent of the sentence and* sock *is the object. A pivot grammar assigns both sentences identical structures, because they consist of the same words in identical order. Other relationships were also common. In the sentence,* sweater chair, *the second word indicates the location of the object named first; thus the sentence is an object-location construction. When Kathryn picked up a hat for a party, she said* party hat, *an instance of an attribute-object construction. All of these sentences are noun-noun sequences, but the use of that description by itself would obscure important semantic distinctions"* (p. 23).

This example illustrates the need for a descriptive grammar to clearly reflect the semantic relationships of an utterance and to differentiate between sentences with identical surface structures but different underlying meanings. Bloom (1970) was one of the first linguists to utilize the concepts of surface and deep structure from transformational grammar in describing early child language. Bloom also pointed out the evidence for determining what the child's intentions are in his early utterances. She proposed that the child's use of appropriate and unvarying word order is evidence of the child's acquisition of semantic relations and that these relations are not just assumed or supplied by the adult interpreter.

SEMANTIC DEVELOPMENT

Increasingly in recent years, the study of child language has moved to include semantics, or meaning. A theory of semantic development has been proposed by Eve Clark (1973) called the **semantic feature hypothesis.** This theory explains that when a child first acquires a word, he has a limited semantic range in his understanding and use of it. Gradually he adds semantic features, perhaps more abstract and not always directly perceptible by adults, until he has acquired the full range of semantic features possessed by the adult speaker.

"For example, let us suppose that the child has learned the word 'dog' (or 'doggie'); however, he only uses one feature to characterize the meaning of this word, so the set of objects that he will put into the category named 'dog' will be larger than the set in the adult category. For instance, he might have characterized the word 'dog' as meaning 'four-legged'; the set of objects referred to as 'dog', therefore, might include cows, sheep, zebras, llamas, dogs and anything else that is four-legged. This feature, four-leggedness, is clearly inadequate to specify the meaning of the word 'dog' in such a way that the child's category will coincide with the adult's (unless the only four-legged creatures the child sees are dogs). However, with the addition of other features, the child will gradually narrow down his initially very general meaning of dog until it means what the adult means. This narrowing-down process will presumably run concurrently with the introduction of new words into the child's vocabulary that take over parts of the overextended semantic domain. To continue with the same example as an illustration, if the child

next acquires the word 'zebra', he must add something to the feature four-legged to keep the meaning of the word distinct from that of 'dog'; he might add any of the following features: hoofs, mane, striped. For the word 'cow,' further specifications might include the sound made (mooing), or other features of shape like horns or udders. At the same time, the child will probably add to the lexical entry for 'dog' things like sound: barking, size: relatively small (in comparison to cows, zebras and llamas), etc. These combinations of features are then used critically, and eventually come to delimit the adult categories'' (Clark, 1973, p. 72).

Another recent approach to the description of child language is the utilization of **case grammar,** as developed by Fillmore (1968). *(TABLE 2.E)* Fillmore demonstrates in this paper that categories more specific than subject and object are needed to describe the adult's use of grammar. It seems that these categories (such as agent, experiencer, objective) are also more appropriate for child language. One of the possible uses of case grammar for teachers of hearing-impaired children is to evaluate what relationships the child is expressing aside from the questions of mode and surface structure problems.

TABLE 2.E Fillmore's case concepts defined and exemplified

FILLMORE'S CASE CONCEPTS DEFINED AND EXEMPLIFIED

CASE NAME	DEFINITION	EXAMPLE (italicized noun is in designated case)
Agentive (*A*)	Typically animate, perceived instigator of action.	*John* opened the door. The door was opened by *John*.
Instrumental (*I*)	The inanimate force or object causally involved in the state or action named by the verb.	The *key* opened the door. John opened the door with the *key*.
Dative (*D*)	The animate being affected by the state or action named by the verb.	*Adam* sees Eve. John murdered *Bill*. John gave the book to *Bill*. *Daddy* has a study.
Factitive (*F*)	The object or being resulting from the state or action named by the verb.	God created *woman*. John built a *table*.
Locative (*L*)	The location or spatial orientation of the state or action named by the verb.	The sweater is on the *chair*. *Chicago* is windy. John walked to *school*.
Objective (*O*)	The semantically most neutral case: anything representable by a noun whose role in the state or action named by the verb depends on the meaning of the verb itself.	Adam sees *Eve*. The *sweater* is on the chair. John opened the *door*.

Source: Roger Brown, *A First Language,* 1973, p. 133.

Roger Brown (1973) evaluates the usefulness of semantically defined cases in describing the utterances of one of his subjects, Adam, at Stage I. He concludes that a case grammar captures many more linguistically significant generalizations and is more useful than the descriptive system of Schlesinger (1971) and Bloom (1973). However, he feels that even using the more semantically aware grammars of Schlesinger, Bloom, and Fillmore, it still is not possible to write a fully explicit grammar of Stage I speech. In fact, Brown (1973) states,

"While case grammar [Fillmore] (1968) deals with more aspects of English than does Schlesinger's grammar of semantic relations, it falls far short of Chomsky's (1965) grammar in this respect. In case grammar as of 1968 there is simply no account given of wh- questions, yes-no questions, the many kinds of negation, the details of conjoining and embedding. All of these things are treated by Chomsky, and so grammars following his lead such as those Bloom has written, start with a great advantage: they lead toward a grammar that represents a large part of adult knowledge" (p. 226).

As discussed earlier in this chapter, we lean heavily on a transformational-generative model of language as the basis of our approach to language development. The developing theories of language acquisition are important to us because the ultimate goal for hearing-impaired children, too, is an adult grammar. To this end, we must be aware of what is learned about the stages of development that the hearing child goes through on his way toward an adult grammar.

SUGGESTED READINGS

COGNITIVE DEVELOPMENT

Almy, M., Chittenden, E., & Miller, P. *Young children's thinking: Studies of some aspects of Piaget's theory.* New York: Teachers College Press, 1967.

Baldwin, A. *Theories of child development.* New York: Wiley & Sons, 1968.

Bronowski, J., & Bellugi, U. Language, name, and concept. *Science,* 1970, p. 168.

Furth, H. *Piaget and knowledge: Theoretical foundations.* Englewood Cliffs, N.J.: Prentice Hall, 1969.

Ginsburg, H. & Opper, S. *Piaget's theory of intellectual development: An introduction.* Englewood Cliffs, N.J.: Prentice Hall, 1969.

LINGUISTIC AND LANGUAGE DEVELOPMENT

Brown, R. *Psycholinguistics: Selected papers.* New York: Free Press, 1970.

Chomsky, N. *Language and mind.* New York: Harcourt, Brace, & Jovanovich, 1968.

Chukovsky, K. *From two to five.* Los Angeles: University of California Press, 1971.

Deese, J. *Psycholinguistics.* Boston: Allyn & Bacon, 1970.

Donaldson, M., & Balfour, G. Less is more: A study of language comprehension in children. *British Journal of Psychology,* 1968, 59. 461–472.

Gleitman, L., Gleitman, H. & Shipley, E. The emergence of the child as grammarian. *Cognition,* 1972, *1,* 137–164.

Opie, I., & Opie, P. *The lore and language of school children.* New York: Oxford University Press, 1959.

ACKNOWLEDGMENTS

QUOTES

Page 8 From *Toward a Theory of Instruction* by Jerome Bruner, 1966. Copyright © 1966 by the President and Fellows of Harvard College. Reprinted by permission of the Belknap Press of Harvard University Press.

Page 11 Page 12 From *Aspects of a Theory of Syntax* by Noam Chomsky, 1965. Copyright © by M.I.T. Press. Reprinted by permission of the publisher.

Page 17 From *Language Development: Structure and Function* by P. Dale, 1976. Copyright © 1976 by Holt, Rinehart, and Winston. Reprinted by permission of the publisher.

Page 17 From "On the Child's Acquisition of Semantics" by E. Clark, in T.E. Moore (Ed), *Cognitive Development and the Acquisition of Language.* Copyright © 1973 Academic Press. Reprinted by permission of the publisher.

FIGURES

Page 6 *Figure 2.1* From *The House at Pooh Corner* by A.A. Milne, 1928. Copyright © 1928 by E.P. Dutton & Co., renewal copyright © 1956 by A.A. Milne. Reprinted by permission of the publisher, E.P. Dutton.

Page 9 *Figure 2.2* From unit prepared by Susan Kondas and Christina Montecalvo, Rhode Island School for the Deaf.

TABLES

Page 15 *Table 2.C,* Page 16 *Table 2.D,* Page 18 *Table 2.E* From *A First Language, The Early Stages* by R. Brown. Copyright © 1973 by Harvard University Press. Reprinted by permission of the President and Fellows of Harvard College.

Chapter 3

The Process of Curriculum Design

A curriculum, by its very nature, demands that it always be in the making. Therefore in discussing curriculum design, we are speaking of the process and only suggesting the product. The process encompasses both theory and method.

The application of theory, or the creation of a framework (curriculum) for teaching and learning, is governed by two elements: the content and the method. Jerome Bruner (1966) cautions:

"One must begin by setting forth the intellectual substance of what is to be taught, else there can be no sense of what challenges and shapes the curiosity of the student. Yet the moment one succumbs to the temptation to 'get across' the subject, at that moment the ingredient of pedagogy is in jeopardy. For it is only in a trivial sense that one gives a course to 'get something across,' merely to impart information. There are better means to that end than teaching. Unless the learner also masters himself, disciplines his taste, deepens his view of the world, the 'something' that is got across is hardly worth the effort of transmission" (p. 73).

The nature of education of the hearing impaired seems to necessitate methods of instruction which are incongruous with the process of learning by discovery. The need to get things across in a straight and unambiguous way is more visibly an issue on the secondary level, but it is just as serious in the elementary grades. However, the dangers of teaching to material rather than teaching to enhance the intellectual powers of the students is a real one and should cause us all to remember that "it avails little to give information that is not asked for" (Bruner, 1966, p. 93).

Bruner, whose views on language were discussed earlier, has also made significant contributions to curriculum design. Among his works on the subject are A Study of Thinking (1967), Toward a Theory of Instruction (1966), The Process of Education (1960), and Beyond the Information Given (1973). In addition, there is the application of many of his curriculum ideas in the controversial program, "Man: A Course of Study" (1966).

His perspectives have provided helpful insight, not so much as to what a curriculum should contain, but rather how it should work. In Bruner's view, a curriculum should be a dynamic process in which the child participates, not a collection of factual information which the child must learn. That is not to say that the acquisition of factual information is unimportant, but that it should not be an end in itself. The real test of learning is what children do with information in the generalizing process rather than the giving back of a series of facts.

The Curriculum Process

Bruner indicates three curriculum processes that should be at work in the classroom. These are the **acquisition of information,** the **transformation of information** and the **evaluation of information.**

The acquisition of information is particularly important for the young child. This process, to which the three levels of representation mentioned earlier (enactive, iconic and symbolic) are related, should be in the mind of the teacher in classroom preparation.

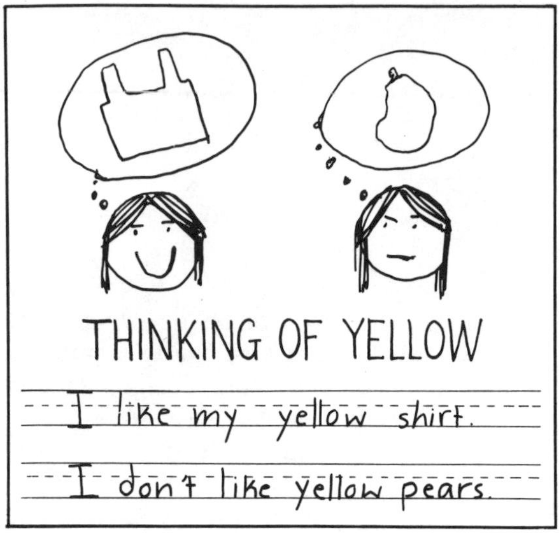

THINKING OF YELLOW

I like my yellow shirt.

I don't like yellow pears.

FIGURE 3.3 Negative categorization

A very common concept discussed in the classroom is that people live in different types of shelters; i.e., house, apartment, town house, etc. The enactive experience is the actual process of visiting the houses and apartments lived in by the children or teachers in the classroom. It is the iconic mode that can help bridge the gap between the experience and language.

Polaroid pictures of the houses or apartments lived in by class members are good visual representations of the real, narrowing the experience to the set of data the language is describing. It is the representation in linguistic (symbolic) form that allows for real internalization to occur and makes for efficiency in recall and generalization.

The transformation of information is an indication that real learning has taken place. Therefore, a curriculum must encourage children to use a generalizing process which goes beyond the mere recognition and comprehension of a particular set of facts. The children must recognize that many other dwellings share the attributes of apartments or houses and can therefore be added to their limited categories. Better still, however, is the identification of certain types of structures that do not fit into the existing categories, creating a need for new categories.

Children are not uncomfortable with what one might call negative categorization and it is often a good thing for a teacher to include negative statements in the presentation of material. (*FIGURE 3.3*)

Another example of negative categorization is the little girl who had red shoes with red shoelaces that eventually broke. Her mother did not have red shoelaces available and instead used red and white striped laces. In describing the situation to a visitor one day, the little girl identified the earlier laces as those which did *not* have white in them, thus classifying the shoelaces with a missing attribute. It may well be that in the learning process, the most interesting criteria used in classifying necessitates that some older categories be identified by what they do not contain.

One of the most satisfying experiences for a teacher is to see students generalize information to new situations, or reform old categories to more adequately handle new material. In a unit of study on the solar system, a class of 7-year-old children were describing some aspects of the planets and used the sentence, "Mars is red." One of the goals of this lesson was to write similes, so the teacher asked the children to think about other things that are red. Their initial response was to point to sweaters and dresses of children in the classroom. While their answers were correct, the teacher pushed a little harder and asked the children to think outside the classroom, to use their imaginations. The results were more satisfying–"leaves in the fall," "party balloons," and for one child the recalling of an experience two years before where she and her mother had made a Japanese flag. Obviously this was a very rich experience, for this child said, "Mars is red like the sun on the flag of Japan." It is this transformation of information that adds excitement to the teaching and learning experience in a classroom.

The evaluation of information, in turn, modifies information previously acquired and transformed. The learning process for any child inevitably results in overgeneralizations and stereotypes. The acquisition of new information should help to modify these overgeneralized categories. This is what is meant by the evaluative process.

Because of the comparative paucity of information available to the hearing-impaired child, it is not unusual for students to go for many years with inappropriate overgeneralizations. For example, one group of students in the Rhode Island School for the Deaf middle school studied Van Gogh and Beethoven as part of a unit on artists and composers. Several years later when these same students were asked a question regarding what was involved in creativity, the students recalled their earlier studies. In focusing more specifically on the question of creativity, a category was formed characterized by, "To be creative is to be neurotic." Having diagnosed this as a problem of overgeneralization, the solution was to do some biographical studies of creative people who were not neurotic.

The ability to evaluate generalizations on the part of both student and teacher is an important part of the curriculum process.

The Spiral Curriculum

Another important contribution by Bruner was his consideration of a spiral component to the curriculum, rather than a curriculum whose units of study are ends in themselves. Traditional curricula are designed to give a "layer effect" to the learning program, such as:

LEVEL 4: Other Communities (cross cultural studies)
LEVEL 3: Community (neighborhood helpers)
LEVEL 2: Family (roles of family members, family activities)
LEVEL 1: Self (personal identification, body parts)

This approach often assumes that what is covered in self concepts, or in family concepts, is a complete and self-contained unit usually unrelated to the units which follow. A spiral curriculum would, in a sense, turn a layer approach on its side so that concepts in all of the categories are spiraled from year to year and, as they become more intricate, begin to interact. (*FIGURE 3.4*)

One of the very difficult aspects of this kind of curriculum design is the identification

A SAMPLE SPIRAL CURRICULUM

Level II	Each person has some role in the family and in society.		People who live in certain environments use the environment for living.
Level I		Various national groups have distinctive physical characteristics.	The world is made up of many countries or nations.
Preschool	Each family has many members.	We live in social groups.	My neighborhood is the area around my home.

FIGURE 3.4 A sample spiral curriculum

of appropriate concepts for each level. Most programs seem fairly comfortable in the early years with studies of self, family, etc. It is important, however, for the secondary level staff to be diagnostic about the knowledge and skills required at their subject level so the appropriate underlying concepts can be dropped (or spiraled) down to meet the conceptual goals of the intermediate and primary departments.

CONCEPT DEVELOPMENT IN THE SPIRAL CURRICULUM

There has been some reference made, from time to time, to concepts. What is suggested here is, rather than a curriculum being designed with vocabulary or factual goals as the desired end, the factual material is utilized to support conceptual statements identified by the teacher. *"The working definition of a concept is the network of inferences that are or may be set into play by an act of categorization"* (Bruner, et al., 1967, p. 224).

Curriculum outlines phrased in conceptual statements will be presented at the end of this chapter. These conceptual statements reflect many of the ideas and units of teaching that have been designed and used successfully by teachers at the Rhode Island School for the Deaf. Because they are conceptual statements, the classroom content used to carry the inferences or data to be categorized may change from year to year, depending on the needs and interests of the children and teachers. (These statements will certainly vary from school to school.) But it cannot be stated too often that the curriculum's ultimate goals are the children's involvement in categorizing processes and the growth of networks of inferences.

The most conceptually sound curriculum needs to be measured by its ability to generate a framework for teaching and learning. It is important that this framework, which will serve as a developmental guideline for organizing a curriculum as well as a practical guide for the presentation of language in the classroom, be consistent with the conceptual basis of the overall approach. This may create some difficulties for the teacher who is required or who chooses to plan utilizing behavioral objectives. However, if one keeps in mind the three processes for learning mentioned earlier - the acquisition of information, the transformation of information, and the evaluation of information - it seems possible to write appropriate behavioral objectives that speak to these three aspects of learning.

While teachers are fairly comfortable with objectives for the acquisition of information, the difficulty occurs in measuring behavior that involves generalizing or learning constraints and categories. The following are examples of objectives written to meet more abstract learning goals.

1. **Acquisition of Information**
   Given two 4-week units of teaching, students shall identify 4 similarities and 4 differences between the family structure of country X and country Y.
2. **Transformation of Information**
   Given that the student can indicate 4 similarities and 4 differences in the family structure of country X and country Y, students shall indicate 4 reasons why the family structure of country Z (new data) is more like that of the family structure in country X or country Y.
3. **Evaluation of Information**
   Given a description of a family structure that does not fit the categories of countries X, Y and Z, students shall indicate one argument as to why the new description does not fit each of countries X, Y and Z.

Language should be seen in this process as the vehicle that represents conceptual categorization and is, in a sense, a measurement of conceptualization itself. A major shift in perspective for the teacher of the deaf is to recognize that for the hearing-impaired child, as well as his hearing peer, language is acquired rather than taught. In the education of the hearing impaired, attention must be given to the language acquisition environment, to the acquisition process itself and, in particular, to the language input and activities that seem necessary to compensate for the sensory deprivation. But this is not to say more language is actually taught. A child functioning with only the language that he or she is taught is a language-disabled child.

A Framework for a Developmental Language Program

The framework for the language development program includes four basic, ordered steps; **exposure, recognition, comprehension,** and **production.** In addition, reading and writing are major components of the overall language program. Reading involves the first three elements (exposure, recognition, and comprehension) and, as will be discussed later, reading and response to literature are types of production as well. Writing is a very special type of production that is integrally related to progress in language and reading. The writing component, in turn, has its own internal organization and parameters that are also developmental in nature.

This framework will be used in this and later chapters to present language goals and language development guidelines and to highlight methods for choosing and presenting language and reading materials. These are guidelines in the widest sense of the word and are not to be used as checklists of skills or structures that teachers are required to teach and students required to learn.

Nor are the steps of the framework to be conceived of as separate entities. A child in the process of acquiring language is involved in all of these steps and components at once.

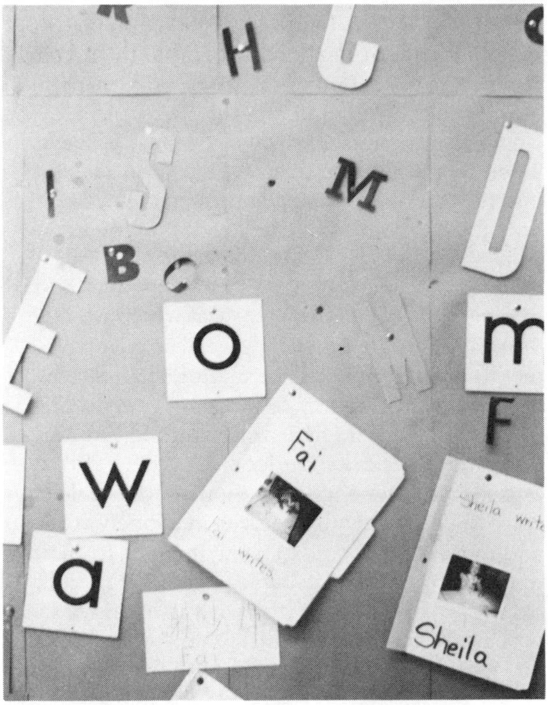

FIGURE 3.5 Beginning exposure to linguistic representation

That is, a child being exposed to complex sentences is perhaps only producing one-word sentences, or a child might be recognizing characterization in a story at a time when he can really only comprehend events in a plot. The elements and components of the language development program, like the learning process they are designed to facilitate, are interrelated.

EXPOSURE

Although there is a general philosophical agreement that hearing-impaired children lack sufficient exposure to language, there seems to be an underlying fear of overexposing the child to too much language input. Consequently, there is a scarcity of language available to children in many classrooms. Only if there is no system for organizing data will overstimulation be a major concern. (*FIGURE 3.5*) One does not learn language without exposure to it; perhaps the last per-

AN EARLY PSYCHOLINGUISTIC EXPERIMENT

The Egyptians before the reign of Psammetichus used to think that of all races in the world they were the most ancient; Psammetichus, however, when he came to the throne, took it into his head to settle this question of priority, and ever since his time the Egyptians have believed that the Phrygians surpass them in antiquity and that they themselves come second. Psammetichus, finding that mere inquiry failed to reveal which was the original race of mankind, devised an ingenious method of determining the matter. He took at random, from an ordinary family, two newly born infants and gave them to a shepherd to be brought up among his flocks, under strict orders that no one should utter a word in their presence. They were to be kept by themselves in a lonely cottage, and the shepherd was to bring in goats from time to time, to see that the babies had enough milk to drink, and to look after them in any other way that was necessary. All these arrangements were made by Psammetichus because he wished to find out what word the children would first utter, once they had grown out of the meaningless baby-talk. The plan succeeded; two years later the shepherd, who during that time had done everything he had been told to do, happened one day to open the door of the cottage and go in, when both children running up to him with hands outstretched, pronounced the word "becos." The first time this occurred the shepherd made no mention of it; but later when he found that every time he visited the children to attend to their needs the same word was constantly repeated by them, he informed his master. Psammetichus ordered the children to be brought to him, and when he himself heard them say "becos" he determined to find out to what language the word belonged. His inquiries revealed that it was the Phrygian word for "bread," and in consideration of this the Egyptians yielded their claims and admitted the superior antiquity of the Phrygians.

FIGURE 3.6 An early psycholinguistic experiment

son to seriously entertain such a notion was King Psammetichus, an early pioneer in the field of language acquisition studies. (*FIGURE 3.6*)

Understanding the hearing-impaired student's need for exposure to a carefully organized language program is an important step in designing a language curriculum. This should help the preschool teacher understand why reading stories to her class, even when her students cannot really understand the structure or all of the vocabulary of that story, is an important part of language exposure. The teacher who recognizes the importance of language exposure will always have books available that are ahead of the reading level of the particular class. For the teacher preparing materials, it is a reminder that not every sentence in a chart is meant to be read, comprehended, understood or spelled.

RECOGNITION

Somewhere between exposure to a wide variety of language experiences and the ability to answer a specific question about a particular sentence of English (which necessitates a comprehension of the information in the sentence and the structure of the question form), there is the glint in the language acquirer's eye, a movement of a hand that says, "I think I've got it!" On many different levels this is a reflection of the recognition of language; the recognition of a name in print, the understanding that a sentence under a cartoon comments on the above visual representation, or the recognition that, even though the hero of a favorite story is in dire straits, he will somehow recover to live happily ever after. Recognition might be defined as an awareness that something perceived has been perceived before.

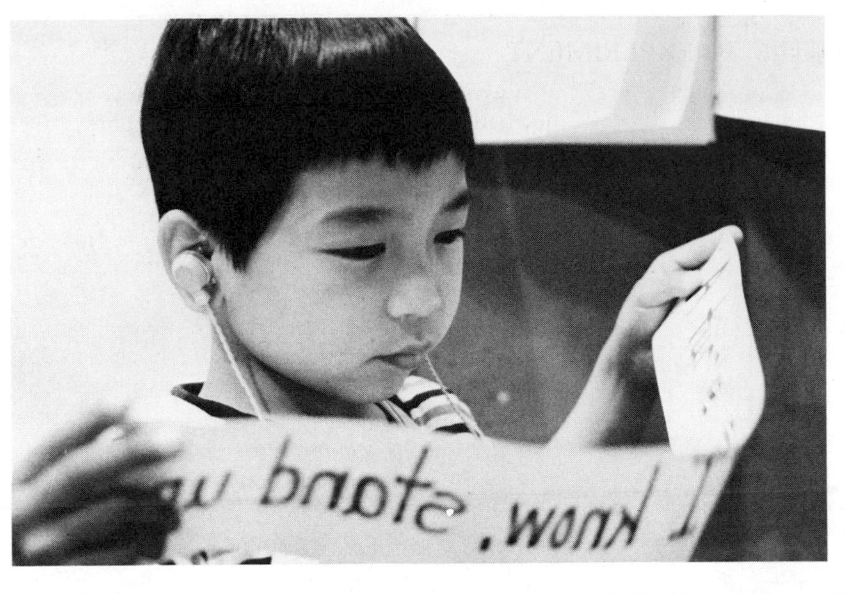

FIGURE 3.7 *For many hearing-impaired children, home and school languages are different.*

The value of identifying recognition as a legitimate part of the comprehension process is that it indicates the child is applying a learning strategy of some kind to a set of data. This, in turn, encourages the teacher to move on to the introduction or exposure of new material to the child, for the more efficient the organizing process becomes, the more understanding should follow.

At a given level, for example, a child may recognize that he is being asked a question but may not comprehend enough of the linguistic structure to really comprehend the question. (Producing the correct response is yet again another task.) Or, for example, in early reading (print-recognition) there is the familiar sight of a child leafing enjoyably through a book that he cannot possibly read. At a secondary level, it is the student recognizing in Art History that the Greeks' striving for perfection has something to do with the word *perfect* but not fully understanding the difference.

One area of increasing concern among educators of the hearing impaired clearly illustrates this recognition stage. There are in many schools for the deaf and other special education programs an increasing number of students from non-English speaking homes. Most of these students enter English-only programs and are expected to comprehend English long before they even recognize that they face a different language in school than at home. (*FIGURE 3.7*)

Recognition also applies to metalinguistic abilities. For example, a group of 11-year-olds easily recognized that a Middle English verse was something like their own language, and they could easily translate most of it. (*FIGURE 3.8*) This is not to say that they understand Middle English, but in the context of a study of the Middle Ages, the recognition of the language difference was important in establishing a conceptual contrast. Similarly, in using "Man: A Course of Study" (1966), the recognition that Eskimos speak a different language was important to the development of concepts relating to differences and similarities in human organization.

This is a poem in Middle English:

Let's feed him
Lat take a cat, and fostre hym
well
wel with milk
tender flesh-meat
And tendre flessh, and make
bed
his couch of silk
let him see mouse
And lat hym seen a mous go
wall
by the wal,
Right now turn away from
Anon he will weyveth milk and
flesh-meat all
flessh and al,
dainty
And every dayntee that is in
house
that hous
Such appetite has eat
Swich appetit hath he to ete a
mouse
mous.

FIGURE 3.8 Recognizing differences in linguistic systems is a useful metalinguistic exercise.

COMPREHENSION

Comprehension is the stage most familiar to language teachers, whether they be teachers of the hearing impaired, teachers of English as a second language, or teachers of other foreign languages. And yet comprehension is most difficult to define as one is not always sure what strategies for understanding language are being used by the child.

Comprehension is the goal of most of our efforts, the heart of language arts. Given an oral or written presentation, do the students really understand the language and content? Do they know who King John was, and what he did, and when and where he did it, and perhaps even why and how? Moreover, can they fill in that information on the right spot on the answer sheet, or in the correct slot on a standardized achievement test?

A student will probably understand or comprehend a given language structure only after long exposure to that particular structure and others that contrast with it, and when he can recognize the general form and function of the structure and only where there is a context and motivation to do so. Comprehension goals, however, often seem measurable only by behavioral goals. Thus, the ability to follow directions can be the be-all and end-all of a language curriculum. But, given a theory that says comprehending language is more than just the ability to act out simple sentences, riddles rather than recipes would be welcome additions to a language curriculum.

WRITING

Writing is an area of linguistic production that is of great concern to teachers and yet is an area where relatively little helpful research is available. In the Rhode Island School for the Deaf Language Curriculum, writing is an important component in the teaching of language and, more importantly, as it functions for the student in the overall language acquisition process. On a very pragmatic level, it is almost always a major part of the classroom learning experience and it is one of the few types of production that teachers feel indicate student mastery of material and content information.

The writing program in the Language Curriculum is constructed on three different but related planes. They are, not in order of importance or development:

The Linguistic Plane: On this plane the relationship between the acquisition of linguistic structures and their appearance in writing is considered. In mapping this relationship, there must be an awareness that the linguistic skills necessary for the mastery of writing may follow some of the developmental steps of general language acquisition but will appear in writing at a later date. *FIGURE 3.9* presents the developmental sequence on this plane.

The Compositional Plane: This plane reflects the cognitive and semantic organizational ability of the student as shown in his writing. It not only includes the order of sentences in a paragraph, but the relationship between a picture and the student's one-word written production. Recent work by Gundlach and Moses (1976) has been most helpful in formulating this part of the Rhode Island School for the Deaf's writing program and a modified version of their developmental steps in composition is presented in *FIGURE 3.10*.

The Functional Plane: This plane focuses on the difference in functions between written language and oral or manual languages. This functional perspective is useful in evaluating the role of writing in the classroom and the actual form of writing assignments that students are asked to respond to.

There are two main classes of writing assignments; teacher-dominated and student-motivated. Letter writing, for example, functions as an independent means of personal expression and yet classroom letter-writing units are often teacher dominated and not a form of self-expression at all. Writing to gain and organize information, as in taking notes (an area, incidentally, where secondary school hearing-impaired students are notoriously poor), is functionally very different from writing a diary.

FIGURE 3.9 Linguistic Parameters in Writing

LINGUISTIC PARAMETERS IN WRITING

I EARLY SCRIBBLING: written language play

II CODE APPROXIMATION: copying, writing, babbling

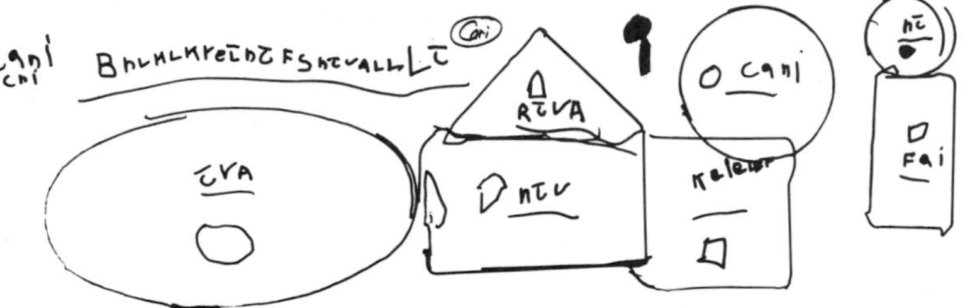

Spontaneous production as produced by a Rhode Island School for the Deaf preschool student

III ACCURATE COPYING AND SOME SPONTANEOUS WRITTEN PRODUCTION: Spontaneous written productions at this stage may look like Levels I and II. Also look for beginnings of phonetic spellings. This level is an indication of **recognition** that writing is a code for the spoken or signed word.

KGlly Kelly Kellr
Clinton rode on a bus.
Clinton rodo on a buk

Cli nt o Nrodeoxq6

Copying and the beginnings of spontaneous production as produced by a Rhode Island School for the Deaf preschool student

IV SPONTANEOUS RECOGNIZABLE PRODUCTIONS: partial words up to simple sentences

June 7, 1976
Riglling
Elepnants

elephanr
Circas
tigen
clow

Beginning recognizable productions, one-word stage, as produced by a first grade hearing student

V SIMPLE SENTENCES (two processes operate within this stage):

1. establishment of a simple sentence grammar
2. variation in simple sentences

I go to Southcocarolina. I haeve goad time in South carolina Water ski. I Learnsail.

Spontaneous productions, simple sentences, as produced by a 9-year-old hearing-impaired student

VI COMPLEX SENTENCES:

1. first expansions: NP complements, simple conjunction, direct discourse, pronominalization
2. simple sentence transformations
   relative clauses
   subordination

shakespeare
shakespeare liked Anne.
Shakespeare liked to write.
Anne said "I want to kiss
shakespeare.
shakespeare and Anne kissed.

First attempts at complexity, infinitive complements, direct discourse, conjunction as produced by an 8-year-old hearing-impaired student

My sister

My sistersplay with me. Her body is thin My sisters stay at home. My sister is busy new york. My sister is worlling in restarant My sister has long hair. My sister has brown hair my sister has a dog. My sister has a baby girl. My sister is coming home Easter. She will give me a present for Easter She work in restaurant before she go to home. She miss me Everyday. She love me.

City Fun

The girl liked to ride the horse, Because The girl feels happy. The people watch the children, Because they care of children. The girl and boy look at horse. The people went to store. The boy looked at little girl. The people has cars. The children like to ride in horse, fireengine. The people feel happy with children. The children wear sweater pant shirt hat shoes and sneaker. Many people walked around sidewalk and crossed the street. The store had restaurant candy land and people has money for ride to children. The people like this place, Because this place is beautiful. I like cars, people and ride horse and fire engine. I feel happy. I looking the picture.

Two samples of writing by the same 11-year-old hearing-impaired girl taken one year apart. The first ("My Sister") indicates that she is functioning in the simple sentence stage, while one year later the writing shows evidence of complexity.

COMPOSITIONAL SKILLS

I Word or sentence with picture: difference between children who draw first and then write and those who illustrate what they have written.

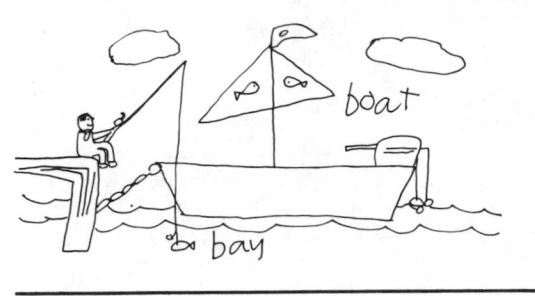

Words with pictures as produced by a 12-year-old hearing-impaired student

II Two to five related but not necessarily ordered sentences.

June 7, 1976
I like The Ringling Bros. Circus. I like The Lions. I like the dog show. I like The clowns show. I Love. trapeze.

Related but unordered sentences as produced by a first grade hearing student

III Two to five related and ordered sentences.

June 7, 1976
The boy went to the Zoo.
He look at the line.
The line got out fo his chge.
The boy ran home.
He LocK his door and went to bed.

Related and ordered sentences as produced by a first grade hearing student

IV Extended written productions: spirals through Levels II and III.

1. two to five related but unordered paragraphs (II)
2. two to five related and ordered paragraphs (III)

In many years ago, the people set up the new subject named English. It made the people to prepared their thoughts to improve themselves in a long time. ago. They used English languages by writings and speakings. The people who lived in Europe moved to America. They used English which carried from their old home to new home. We used English alot so we projected ourselves into higher level in our minds. English used us to know how to write and how to speak the way English was. English was the hardest subject in the world because it had every-one word with many different meanings. The people studied English very hard to understand the way it was.

Extended written production as produced by a high school senior from the Rhode Island School for the Deaf

FIGURE 3.10 Compositional Skills

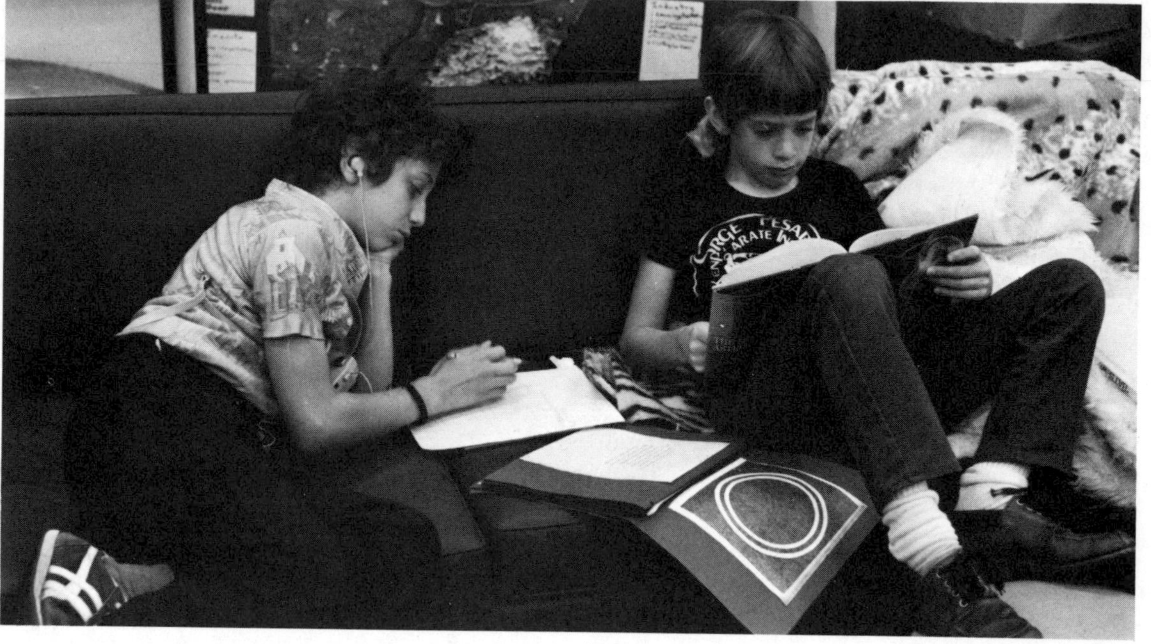

Figure 3.11

The Role of Reading and Literature in Curriculum

Because content within conceptual statements will alter in classrooms from year to year, so will the content of the reading material alter. For this reason the network of inferences made by readers is not governed by any one specific story or group of stories. Therefore the elements of literature must be introduced at a young age and spiraled into an overall curriculum. There has too often been a dichotomy between teaching reading and language skills on one hand, and expecting significant personal growth and involvement through literature on the other.

Trying to teach reading skills alone brings about a preoccupation with vocabulary, a preponderance in dealing with things concrete rather than symbolic or abstract, and finally a repeatedly inefficient method of separating reading, writing, and literature. The teaching of reading should be directed toward developing all the mechanical skills: phonics, word skills and comprehension strategies, as well as developing all the student's abilities to use reading as a means of thinking and experiencing. This ability depends heavily upon the experience of both the reader and the writer.

The potentials of language, particularly in literature, go far beyond simple communication. Reading and literature as parts of curriculum design provide space in which personal response protects against the totally experience-based approach. This approach ignores one major truth: *"How difficult it is for human beings to see generality in what has become familiar"* (Bruner, 1966, p. 94).

Pupils need reading experiences that develop depth of insight. Unless they do considerable reading that is spontaneous and enjoyable, they are not likely to have sufficient practice in reading to develop the skills necessary for a greater appreciation of literature. Kenneth Koch, in Rose, Where Did You Get That Red? (1973), shows how literature must be a dynamic, liberating experience in which the child's own reading and writing complement each other.

Based on his experience with teaching children to write poetry, Koch argues that an early exposure to literature will allow children to find materials they like. Interesting is Koch's comment that most of the poetry found in children's anthologies or readers is not as valuable as the poetry created by the children themselves. Koch feels that there is a *"condescension toward children's minds and abilities in regard to poetry in almost every elementary text . . ."* (p. 7). In the education of the hearing impaired, this attitude is often exhibited, not only in relation to poetry, but also in relation to the entire discipline of literature.

An appreciation of literature comes from an increasing sense of relatedness between literature and life. There must be a progression from understanding the simplest levels of literal meaning to grasping abstract levels of symbolization and inference. Elements of description, imagery, metaphor, allegory or irony must be made available to the student as well. These are skills that have to be mastered (at some point) if meaningful interaction between reader and text is to be achieved.

A child can respond initially to literature, and this response is valid. However, if the quality of his response is not refined, if he does not bring new information to the text as well as retain the old, literature will not have fulfilled its purpose. There are, as Rosenheim states, *"degrees of pleasure that are largely determined by the degree of affirmative intellectual energy a reader is willing to invest"* (in Egoff et al., 1969, p. 19).

It seems essential that a reading curriculum, as with curriculum development in general, be modeled after Bruner's spiral pattern–building complex skills on the mastery of simpler ones. This would assume, for instance, that a student does not begin with T. S. Eliots' "The Love Song of J. Alfred Prufrock," nor reach the age of 16 before he is exposed to metaphor. Bruner states:

". . . There is an appropriate version of any skill or knowledge that may be imparted at whatever age one wishes to begin teaching–however preparatory the version may be. The choice of the earlier version is based upon what it is hoping to cumulate. The deepening and enrichment of this earlier understanding is again a source of reward for intellectual labors" (Bruner, 1966, p. 35).

Literature can be used to exploit the reader's curiosity and to challenge his language sense. The characters and events should summon up what the reader knows about people and things and somehow strengthen his understanding of human nature. Perhaps most importantly, the reading process should provide him with a sense of active encounter and achievement.

Traditional reaction has been to accept what is being said about the vitality of literature and yet, because of language and reading delay, discount its possibilities in the curriculum for the hearing impaired. The literature studied by hearing-impaired children is usually restricted to juvenile texts and rewrites. These texts lack the fundamental appeal of good literature: a combination of authenticity and wonder of life through language.

Kenneth Koch (1973) addresses this point in regard to teaching poetry. *"I wasn't put off by some of the difficulties teachers are often bothered by–unfamiliar words and difficult syntax, for example, and allusions to unfamiliar things. My students learned new words and new concepts in order to play a new game, or to enable them to understand science fiction or comics, or on TV, so why not for poetry?"* (p. 10). Koch does admit that there are obviously passages within a poem which are going to remain obscure. But he also feels that to reject every poem containing an obscurity would be to reject too many good things in literature.

Koch expresses the need for literature to be more than just an "ornament," more than background music or a nice break from the classroom day. He is revolted by the childishness of so much of the literature used for young people; literature which is likely to turn children away from appreciating poetry.

The cloyingly sweet and troublefree view of life, *"conspires against a child's development and literature itself"* (p. 13). This concern is also restated in an article by Penelope Farmer (1972) on children's literature. She states that children take from books what they most need at that particular time, *". . . . from wish fulfillment at the lowest level, upwards to the pointing and even partial resolving of the most complex of subconscious dilemmas"* (p. 37).

Literature is an important part of the curriculum and spirals into larger and larger realms as the language and conceptual abilities of the students grow. Literature is not seen as a separate area, but rather as an integral part of the language and reading program. In addition, the potentials of literature in affecting the personal growth of students are unlimited and this alone is justification for its prominence in the curriculum.

SUGGESTED READINGS

CURRICULUM DESIGN

Bruner, J.S. *Contemporary approaches to cognition: A symposium held at the University of Colorado.* Cambridge, MA: Harvard University Press, 1964.

Bruner, J.S. *The relevance of education.* New York: Norton Press, 1971.

Kogan, M. (Ed). *Informal schools in Britain today.* New York: Citation Press, 1972.

Taylor, P., Reid, W., & Kelly, P. (Eds). *Journal of Curriculum Studies.* Glasgow: Collins Educational Press, 1968.

ACKNOWLEDGMENTS

FIGURES

Page 26 *Figure 3.6* From Herodotus, *The Histories* translated by Aubrey de Selincourt (Penguin Classic), 1954, p. 102–103. Copyright © 1954 by the Estate of Aubrey de Selincourt. Reprinted by permission of Penguin Books, Ltd.

Page 27 *Figure 3.7* Photograph courtesy of Ira Garber.

Page 28 *Figure 3.8* From unit prepared by David Vryhof, Rhode Island School for the Deaf.

Page 29 *Figure 3.9* Writing samples courtesy of Margaret Antoniou, Judy Tartaglia, Mary Weiner, and Lois Fain, Rhode Island School for the Deaf; Donna Jarett, Martin Luther King School.

Page 31 *Figure 3.10* Writing samples courtesy of Elizabeth Dogan, Rhode Island School for the Deaf; Donna Jarett, Martin Luther King School.

Page 32 *Figure 3.11* Photograph courtesy of Ira Garber.

Page 44 *Figure 3.14* From unit on Japan prepared by Marilyn Cooney, Rhode Island School for the Deaf; From unit on Africa prepared by Mary Weiner, Rhode Island School for the Deaf. Photograph courtesy of Ira Garber.

Page 50 *Figure 3.15* Analysis sample from a language unit prepared by Barbara Simon, Rhode Island School for the Deaf.

QUOTES

Page 21
Page 33 From *Toward a Theory of Instruction* by Jerome Bruner, 1966. Copyright © 1966 by the President and Fellows of Harvard College. Reprinted by permission of the Belknap Press of Harvard University Press.

The following summarizes the sequence of themes and language skills currently in use at the Rhode Island School for the Deaf. This outline presents only the skeleton of the developmental language and learning curriculum and variation should be expected. Levels are exemplified by the conceptual outlines that follow this thematic and linguistic outline.

PRESCHOOL/LOWER SCHOOL/MIDDLE SCHOOL CURRICULUM OUTLINE

LEVEL	THEMATIC OUTLINE	NEW LANGUAGE SKILLS
Preschool I *3–5 years*	A. The child in the family and at school	Recognition of sentence types Basic word order Pronominalization within sentences
Preschool II *5–6 years*	B. The family in society	Conjoining Question formation
Lower School I *6–7 years*	A. The child and family in other societies B. Personal awareness (physical, psychological, emotional)	Simple sentence grammar Simple conjunction Infinitive NP Movable adverbs
Lower School II *7–8 years*	A. The environment in which people live B. Family roles	Subordination - adverb clause Question forms
Lower School III *8–9 years*	A. The history of peoples and societies B. Social roles	Pronominalization across sentences Nonmovable adverbs
Lower School IV *9–10 years*	A. Racial origins and cultural expression B. The movement of peoples and cultures	Relational conjunction Dative
Middle School I *10–11 years*	Cultural interaction: Changes that occur when cultures interact with each other	Subordination-relative clause Passive voice
Middle School II *11–12 years*	The human condition: People need to respond to situations and events	*How/why* questions *If/then* clauses
Middle School III *12–13 years*	The riddle of the past: The various ways that we learn about people in other times	NP complements Relative clause reduction Topicalization
Middle School IV *13–14 years*	Being human: Some factors that make people distinctively human	Various deletions Nominalization

The following are conceptual outlines and possible topics for the various levels of the language and learning curriculum. Topics will most likely vary from school to school.

LEVEL: Preschool I and II
Thematic Outline
A. The child in the family and at school
B. The family in society

CONCEPTUAL STATEMENTS

A. *Concepts of Self*
1. People have personal names.
2. People have family names.
3. All people share certain physical characteristics.
4. All people have certain physical needs: food, shelter, clothing.
5. All people have certain feelings.

B. *Concepts of Social Relationships*
1. Each family has many members.
2. Each member of the family has different characteristics.
3. Each member of the family has some characteristics in common with the other members.
4. All family members have first and last names.
5. Each member has a different job.
6. People who live nearby are our neighbors.
7. People in our school have different jobs.
8. Other people in our neighborhood help the people who live there in various ways.
9. We live in social groups.

C. *Concepts of Physical Environment*
1. A person's home is where he lives.
2. My neighborhood is the area right around my home.
3. School is where teachers help children to learn many things.
4. The community is a large place and encompasses many neighborhoods.
5. Many people in the community participate together in different activities.
6. There are different kinds of communities.
7. People live in different parts of the world.

POSSIBLE TOPICS

—Most of the activities of the preschool level involve the beginnings of basic understandings by the child as a member of a family and as a member of society.
—Units involving naming or identification of universal physical characteristics can involve stories that reinforce these concepts.
—Units of food, shelter and clothing are popular at the preschool level.
—In studying feelings it is important that feelings that do not appear on the face, such as loneliness, be included.

LEVEL: Lower School I (6-7 years)
Thematic Outline
A. The child and family in other societies

CONCEPTUAL STATEMENTS

1. The world is made up of many countries or nations.
2. Various national groups have distinctive physical characteristics.
3. All people use language, but not all languages are the same.
4. All people eat food. Different national groups eat different foods.
5. Most people wear clothing, but different national groups have distinctive clothing.
6. Play is a part of most people's life style, but games are often different from nation to nation.
7. Most people have religious beliefs, but there are different beliefs and means of expression.
8. Most national groups celebrate through festivities, but *what* is celebrated and *how* are often distinctive.
9. Although most communities have a family structure, the roles of family members often differ from community to community.

POSSIBLE TOPICS

—Because of the age of the children it is probable that the contrast between people is often noticed and tends to lead to overgeneralization. This overgeneralization will be modified by later studies in the curriculum.

—There are underlying implications in the outline, however, that should be emphasized whenever possible, (i.e., *All* people eat food, but, all people do not necessarily eat the same food. *All* people use language, but all people do not use the same language. Almost all people wear clothing, but all people do not wear the same clothing.) The choice as to the societies chosen is somewhat arbitrary. One teacher spent four weeks each on some of the special events of the calendar.

January	Switzerland (Winter)
February	Japan
March	Ireland (St. Patrick's Day)
April	Holland
May	Egypt

—If the choice is to cover a lesser number of countries, then to be an effective organizing process there should be at least three countries studied, each with enough distinctiveness for contrast and comparison purposes.

LEVEL: Lower School I (6-7 years)
Thematic Outline
B. Personal awareness: Physical, social, psychological, emotional

CONCEPTUAL STATEMENTS

1. The child has developing needs and abilities in the areas of physical, social, intellectual and emotional growth.
2. Growth enlarges the child's capacity but increases the risks.
   a) Children grow physically.
      1. grow taller
         grow wider
         grow heavier
      2. parts grow independently
         hair grows
         finger and toenails grow
      3. people grow stronger
         people grow older
   b) Children grow socially.
      1. as children grow they move from isolation to group interaction which means learning turn-taking, social rules, etc.
   c) As children grow they become more knowledgeable.
      1. the senses are used to organize the world
      2. language is used to organize the world
   d) Children have new experiences in physical, social and intellectual growth.
      1. create challenges to a child's feelings about self and others
      2. need to grow on an emotional level

POSSIBLE TOPICS

—Teachers are most probably comfortable describing the physical aspects of growth, which can involve so much enactive, iconic and symbolic processing.
—It is important that children develop concepts of growth in other areas as well.
—The use of games and turn-taking can be used to help describe the interaction here.
—The Brute Family has been used very successfully to introduce behavior patterns.
—The utilization of sense experiences can be used very effectively, enabling the use of linking verbs and adjectives to be expanded. It is valuable to use the adjectives in contrast.

tastes	sour
	sweet
looks	ugly
	beautiful
feels	soft
	hard
	rough
smells	awful
	nice
sounds	loud
	soft

The role of language can be used to describe, tell, etc.
—It is important that the adjectives which describe the emotions are introduced. This perhaps can be best done by the use of stories that describe those feelings, such as "The Ugly Duckling."

LEVEL: Lower School II (7-8 years)
Thematic Outline:
A. The environment in which people live

CONCEPTUAL STATEMENTS

1. Environmental features are often related to geographical factors.
2. Plants are specific to certain kinds of environments.
3. Animals are specific to certain kinds of environments and they feed on the plants or animals of the area.
4. People who live in these environments use the environment for living.
   a) They eat plants and animals for food.
   b) They use plants and animals for shelter, clothing and tools.
5. Some aspects of the environment are directly useful (i.e., the seasons, the climate, the sun, the moon).
6. People who live in these environments regard the factors in the environment as very important.
   a) They celebrate seasons and harvests.
   b) They create myths about features in the environment.

POSSIBLE TOPICS

—A contrast can be meaningfully established here between *jungles* and *deserts* or between *arctic* and *temperate* and *tropical* zones. The actual studies can involve Africa, South America, the Arctic, Australia, India or the U.S.A. The contrast can be carried into a study of the herbage of the environments. This is also an opportunity to introduce herbivorous/carnivorous animal categories.
—Kipling's "Jungle Stories" are useful to utilize here.
—Children of this age enjoy studies of the solar system and the seasons.
—A goal of this study is to see the interaction between people and the plants, animals and terrain of the environment. The battle with the elements is a widespread myth and the role of the taboo can be introduced here.

LEVEL: Lower School II (7-8 years)
Thematic Outline
B. Family Roles

CONCEPTUAL STATEMENTS

1. Each person has some role in the family and the society.
2. Our roles are related to each other in the family.
3. Our roles are often related to the influence of the society in which we live.
4. Roles often mean responsibilities.
5. When people don't live up to their responsibilities, problems occur.
6. When the family structure breaks down, people have to assume new roles.
7. Special needs in the family mean new roles and responsibilities for people. (i.e., A handicapped child means new responsibilities for all the other members of the family.)
8. When new responsibilities are added, there is often less time, money or opportunity to do other things.

POSSIBLE TOPICS

—It is important for the child to experiment with many roles. By this we mean letting him or her play at being different people, different things, for it is the ability to *take the role of other people* that makes the human animal a social being. Prejudice is based on an inability to imagine how the world looks to the other fellow.
—As with many other topics at this stage some of these concepts might best be introduced through stories such as "The Ugly Duckling."
—Because it is not unusual for children to come from one parent families, the curriculum needs to discuss the disintegration of the family as well as the structure.
—As role understanding involves the ability of the person to see things from someone else's point of view, this is a good time to discuss, not only hearing loss, but its effect on the whole family.

LEVEL: Lower School III (8-9 years)
Thematic Outline
A. The history of peoples and societies

CONCEPTUAL STATEMENTS

1. History involves the study of great civilizations.
   a) Great civilizations are identified by their:
      1. dominance in world affairs.
      2. technological development.
      3. contributions through art forms.
      4. commitment to great ideas that have solidified or motivated the society.
2. History involves the study of great ideas.
   a) Ideas are shared by people.
   b) Ideas are represented in many forms—fable, legend, art, music.
   c) Great ideas are often preserved in monuments, books, poetry, music, legends.
3. History involves the study of great people.
   a) People have played important roles in the development of great civilizations.
   b) People play important roles in spreading ideas—scholars, artists, inventors, philosophers, scientists.

POSSIBLE TOPICS

—The goal of this study is not to do an extensive historical survey but to develop a sense for historical perspective and the concept that one can view history as an interaction of great ideas and great people.
—Children are interested in biography and enjoy the materials related to the stories.
—The particular eras and civilizations studied are somewhat arbitrary and should not be allowed to bog down in great detail - that will come later.

LEVEL: Lower School III (8-9 years)
Thematic Outline
B. Social roles

CONCEPTUAL STATEMENTS

1. Roles for people are often determined by the needs of a family (i.e. rural vs. technological societies).
2. The needs of the family are often interwoven with the needs of the society in which it lives.
3. The more complex the society, the greater the interdependence of roles.
4. The simpler the environment, the clearer role definition is.
5. Some roles are related to:
   a. specific tasks (i.e., farmers, millers, craftsmen).
   b. supportive tasks (i.e., preachers, school teachers).
   c. enriching tasks (i.e., musicians, artists, composers).

POSSIBLE TOPICS

—As some studies are being done with a historic perspective, it might be useful to study the roles of people in earlier communities such as:
  The Early American Community
  The Medieval Town
and contrast the roles with those in our society building on concepts of social relationships and physical environments of the preschool.
—One teacher rewrote *A Christmas Carol* and studied the roles of various people to great effect.
—There is also good opportunity for biography in this study.

LEVEL: Lower School IV (9-10 years)
Thematic Outline
A. Racial origins and cultural expression

CONCEPTUAL STATEMENTS

1. Racial groups can often be identified by physical characteristics.
2. Major racial groups often share similar cultural factors.
3. Distinctive cultural factors are often seen in family and social structure.
4. Cultural distinctions are often expressed in various art forms.
5. Art forms, myths and rituals enable a society to share and reaffirm its culture.
6. Art forms, myths and rituals enable a society to hand on its culture to a new generation.

POSSIBLE TOPICS

—Many of these concepts are extensions of those studied in Lower School I, The Child and Family in Other Societies (p 37).
—Studies of cultural expressions such as oriental art, music, or aboriginal rituals need to be extended to see the universal issues of initiation, educational processes, and the assuming of responsibilities.

LEVEL: Lower School IV (9-10 years)
Thematic Outline
B. The movement of peoples and cultures

CONCEPTUAL STATEMENTS

1. Many countries are made up of a variety of people from different cultural backgrounds.
2. People move for a variety of reasons.
   a) famine
   b) persecution
   c) war
   d) opportunity
3. When people migrate they take many of their cultural distinctions with them.
4. Although many factors will change in time, some remain.

POSSIBLE TOPICS

—A very effective activity is to collect data from the families of children in the school or class. When did their ancestors come to this country? Why did they come? What were their names before they came?
—By putting pins on the map indicating areas from which people came and by studying the corresponding dates one can often see the waves of immigration.

LEVEL: Middle School I (10-11 years)
Thematic Outline
Cultural interaction: Changes occur when cultures interact with each other

CONCEPTUAL STATEMENTS

1. Cultures come into contact for various reasons:
   a) war
   b) persecution
   c) poverty
   d) opportunity
2. When cultures come into contact, change occurs
   a) in language.
   b) in art forms.
   c) in social structure.
3. Individuals and families are affected by intercultural contact.
   a) People must often work together to survive.
   b) Children often have different value systems than their parents.
   c) Some people become leaders.
   d) People express their feelings in art forms.

POSSIBLE TOPICS

—The vehicles that illustrate intercultural contact are many. Specific studies of each reason for contact can be studied, such as the Irish immigration, Russian history (from the Czars to immigration including Fiddler on the Roof) or the disintegration of the Incan empire.
—Many interesting examples of changes in language and art forms that indicate intercultural contact are available.
—In the history of the English language for example, some words came from the French as a result of the Norman conquest and yet many Saxon words survived for very pragmatic reasons.
—The third set of concepts might include the following, depending on the abilities of the students:

sociological studies
biography
literature

LEVEL: Middle School II (11-12 years)
Thematic Outline
The human condition: People must respond to situations and events.

CONCEPTUAL STATEMENTS

1. There are events that occur in every person's life.
   a) life
   b) growth
   c) social interaction
   d) success and failure
   e) death
2. People must respond to these events.
   a) They celebrate formally.
   b) They respond emotionally.
3. Some situations do not occur in all people's experiences.
   a) riches or poverty
   b) uprooting
   c) great success
   d) tragedy
4. People must respond to the above events.

POSSIBLE TOPICS

—A basic introduction to the life cycle can be accomplished here, although the actual cycle itself might be better dealt with at Level IV.
—Growth can include a specific study of growth itself, especially as these students are entering adolescence.
—A more symbolic study can be done through songs, such as "Puff the Magic Dragon" or a more intense study of aging through Simon and Garfunkels' "Bookends"
—The way in which people formally respond to these events can include myth (especially initiation), song and ritual.
—Biography, literature and song can be used successfully to illustrate numbers 3 and 4 of the conceptual statements.
—A historical study such as the Middle Ages and the Renaissance enables one vehicle to cover all the conceptual statements involved.

LEVEL: Middle School III (12-13 years)
Thematic Outline
The riddle of the past: There are various ways that we learn about people in other times.

CONCEPTUAL STATEMENTS

1. We learn about people in the past through:
   a) archaeology.
   b) people's written records.
   c) official records.
   d) art forms.
2. People study these items.
   a) archaeologists
   b) historians
   c) linguists
   d) anthropologists
3. There are specific ways in which studies are carried out.

POSSIBLE TOPICS

—Although the conceptual statements are somewhat simple in this topic, the studies involve one conceptual statement which is important for later studies in both the middle and upper schools.
—For instance, it is important not only to be able to read language but to know what a journal, or a history book, or Town Hall records are for.
—The opportunity to do some work on career education is possible here, as well as some biographical studies of outstanding scholars.
—Section 3 of the conceptual statements lends itself to some very specific "hands on" activities including:
  an archaeological dig.
  studying an old family tree using records and newspapers.
  studying the Rosetta stone (replica available through Alva replicas).
  classifying various collections such as bottles and artifacts.

LEVEL: Middle School IV (13-14 years)
Thematic Outline
Being human: There are some factors that make people distinctively human.

CONCEPTUAL STATEMENTS

1. All people share certain physical and mental characteristics.
2. All people share certain emotional characteristics.
3. All people share certain spiritual characteristics.
4. People share certain needs related to these characteristics.
5. People share certain wants related to these characteristics.
6. Some of the factors are hereditary and innate.
7. Some of the factors are learned.

POSSIBLE TOPICS

—The important emphasis in this outline is not what is different about people or other countries, nations or racial groups, but what is shared or universal.
—A helpful commercial project is "Man: A Course of Study" (Curriculum Development Associates) which addresses the question: What is human about being human?

The following are samples of unit plans developed out of the conceptual outlines for lower school. The unit plan indicates various subject areas that are integrated into the unit planning process.

A UNIT PLAN ON JAPAN FOR LOWER SCHOOL I

INTRODUCTION

The children were already familiar with the world map and globe and the location of America and Switzerland. The flag of Japan was placed on the map and the language story was told about a girl who lived in Japan. Pictures of the country and people were shown and discussed and placed on the bulletin board. A series of slides was then given showing Japanese people, costumes, schools, homes, temples and customs. Books with stories about Japanese children, magazines and filmstrips from the library were also used periodically.

LANGUAGE STORIES

1. Meho in Japan

Meho lived in Japan.
She walked to school.
All the children wore school uniforms.
After school, Meho played.
Mother said, "It's time for supper."
Meho ate rice.
She slept on the floor.

2. Rice and Tea

We made rice and tea.
Louis poured water into the pan.
Jeff stirred the rice.
The water boiled.
Michael said, "Be careful!"
Everyone drank tea.
Oops! The rice fell off the chopsticks.
Paulette ate a lot!
Wendy didn't like it!

3. A Party

Meho opened a letter.
It said, "Come to a party."
Meho wore a long dress.
She put flowers in her hair.
Meho looked beautiful!
Meho went to the party.
The party was full!
(This story was done during the week of Valentines Day, so a story was chosen which related to holidays and special occasions in preparation for our own party.)

Each story was told using picture sequence cards and sentence strips. Each story was then printed on a chart without pictures. One story was introduced each week. Children matched sentences to pictures and vice versa, and attempted verbal production of sentences. Children also identified sentences on the chart by using both auditory and lipreading skills alone. Copies of the stories were dittoed in book form for the children to take home and read to their parents. Children also drew illustrations of the stories and printed sentences to make their own book for the classroom.

RELATED ACTIVITIES

Art. During class the children made fans and Japanese lanterns with which they decorated the classroom. In the art room the children painted and assembled a large cardboard temple with a roof of chicken wire stuffed with paper flowers. The temple was large enough for all the children to get inside. The children also made a type of paddle in art and played a Japanese game similar to badminton. A Japanese student from a nearby university introduced the children to origami.

A Japanese kimono, shoes, fans, umbrellas and hats were obtained for display in the classroom. Each child dressed in Japanese clothes and had his picture taken for our school scrapbook. Pictures were taken of all the related experiences and put in the book with one sentence under each for the children to read during free time.

The children made rice and tea in the classroom and ate at a low table while sitting on the floor Japanese style (kneeling with shoes off and feet crossed). They ate with chopsticks which they got to take home. (Most of the children used them again at home to eat their evening meal.)

Each child had his name printed in Japanese on the bulletin board. The children practiced printing their names in Japanese.

Each child colored and cut out a Japanese flag and compared it to other flags as to color and design. One girl made a flag at home by sewing a red circle to a white piece of cloth.

The unit ended with a trip to a Japanese restaurant. Each child sampled many different Japanese foods. They ate with chopsticks while sitting on the floor, Japanese style.
They also got to see many Japanese people. A photographer was there from the local paper and the picture of the children eating appeared in the paper the following day.

A SAMPLE UNIT PLAN ON AFRICA FOR LOWER SCHOOL II

ASSUMED CONCEPTS

People in other countries have unique customs.

Primitive man depends on his environment directly.

Some animals have social structures.

Species of animals differ according to geography.

NEW CONCEPTS

Primitive society still exists.

Modern civilization is found in close proximity to these primitive groups.

Some wildlife is threatened.

Some animals have a highly developed social structure similar to man's.

Some animals are herbivorous and some are carnivorous.

UNIT OUTLINE

I. The geography of Africa
II. The animals of Africa
III. The people of Africa

SUBJECT SKILLS

Language/Reading

—Using the Tuareg Alphabet to write names, short sentences, and short stories such as "Anansi the Spider."

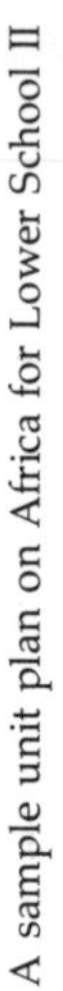

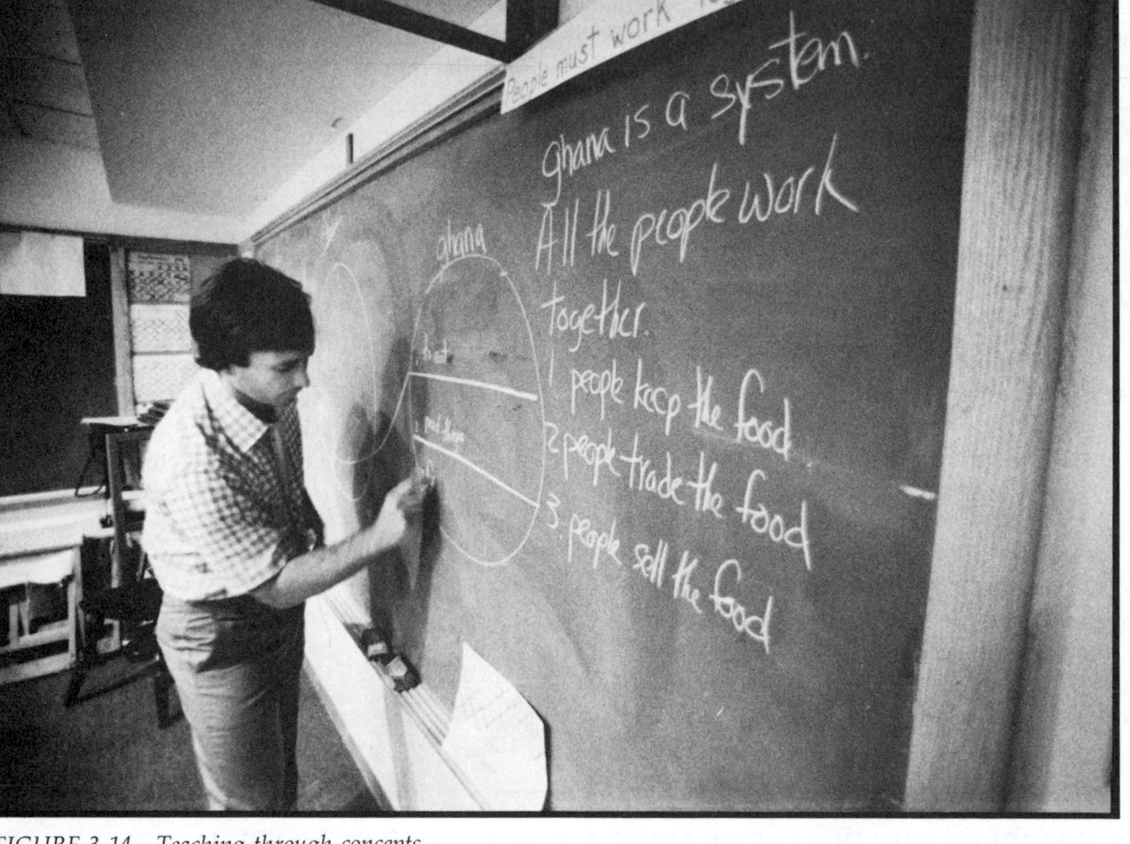
People must work
Ghana is a system.
All the people work
together.
1 people keep the food
2 people trade the food
3. people sell the food
ghana

FIGURE 3.14 Teaching through concepts.

Social Studies

—Different cultures within Africa and how they cope with their environment.

The Tuaregs—Sahara Desert
The Bushmen—Kalahari Desert
West Africans—Fishermen
East Africans—Farmers
Pygmies—Congo, Jungle
Zulus—South Africa

Math

—Map work—new terms; North, South, East, West. Word problems using new language from this unit.
—Counting to 10 in Swahili

Science

—The animals of Africa—herbivorous vs. carnivorous

their dependence on each other
their relation to geography
safaris and hunting
zoos and animal capture
baboon society in detail, dominant male leader, rearing of the young, etc. . .
the equator

Art

—Slides from RISD Museum
—Making African masks in art class

Music

—Playing an African tune on melodicas.
—Listening to African music on records.

The following are outlines of the language development program at the Rhode Island School for the Deaf, preschool through high school. These are intended as guidelines for language planning and goal setting and not as fixed objectives to be met in a finite period of time. The guidelines are presented in the Exposure, Recognition, Comprehension, and Production framework, with additional guidelines in Reading and Writing.

LANGUAGE DEVELOPMENT OUTLINE: Preschool Through Kindergarten

EXPOSURE

1. Egocentric/repetitive chart stories representing classroom experiences. By the end of the second year, students should be exposed to nonegocentric/nonrepetitive chart stories.
2. Simple sentences, especially patterns one and two. Adverbials should be frequently added to pattern one sentences. By the end of the second year, students should have been exposed to all five basic sentence patterns.
3. Other syntactic categories for exposure
   a) negation
   b) *do* as an auxiliary
   c) prepositional phrases
   d) personal pronouns, especially in object position
   e) question types/interrogatives
      i *who* and *what* questions about all patterns
      ii *where* and *when* questions where appropriate
      iii *did . . . do* questions about verbs in patterns one and two
4. Functional and affective language
   a) egocentric expressions: likes to, wants to, can
   b) sentence types: declarative, interrogative, imperative
   c) turn-taking language routines
   d) language-play activities

COMPREHENSION/RECOGNITION

1. Sentence types, recognition by intonation
   a) imperatives
   b) interrogatives
   c) declaratives
2. Sentence patterns one and two
   a) *who* questions about patterns one and two
   b) *what* questions about patterns one and two
   c) some *when* and *where* questions about adverbials in pattern one sentences.
3. Lexicon: nouns and verbs growing out of classroom experiences that are described in language experience charts.
4. Functional and affective language
   a) own name
   b) classmates' names
   c) beginning of social greeting system
5. Sentence form (recognition only)
   a) in sentence strip form
   b) in conversation
6. Different functions of language (recognition only)
   a) story form (language for fun)
   b) information or experience story (language for information)
7. By the end of the second year there should be a recognition of all sentence patterns although comprehension may only extend through patterns one and two.

PRODUCTION

1. Syntactic goals: In this stage the child may progress through the following sequence:
   a) holophrastic/telegraphic
   b) ordered-two word sentences (by end of 1st year)
   c) three- to five-word sentences, although word order may break down in longer sentences
2. Other syntactic goals
   a) beginning of question formation: use of *who* or *what* with another noun or verb
   b) beginning use of adverbials
   c) meaningful use of S-V-O (subject-verb-object) word order
3. Functional and social language
   a) own name
   b) classmates' names
   c) family members
   d) language play
   e) initiation of communication

READING/PRINT RECOGNITION

1. Printed symbols
2. Classroom directions
3. Own name, names of classmates
4. Verbs, especially from repetitive charts
5. Nouns: recognition of common classroom names, animals, etc.
6. Sentence form as a whole
7. Recognition of print as meaningful and ordered
8. Book form (recognition)

WRITING (in this stage, writing may precede reading)

1. Scribbling
2. Code approximation
3. By end of second year, can write own name
4. Fairly accurate copying, preserving sentence form by end of second year
5. Awareness that letters and writing are part of a meaningful system
6. Written language play
7. Beginning functional use of writing

LANGUAGE DEVELOPMENT OUTLINE: The Simple Sentence Stage

EXPOSURE

1. Syntactic considerations
   a) all five sentence patterns
   b) narrative language
      i sequential adverbs
      ii prepositional phrases
      iii adverbial clauses
   c) descriptive language
      i sentence pattern three
      ii simile and metaphor
   d) infinitive complements in object position (*likes to, wants to*)
   e) some auxiliary verbs
   f) different tenses in context
   g) different forms of negation
   h) expanded pronoun system (e.g., possesives)
   i) conjunction, especially in object position
   j) simple sentence conjunction
   k) question formation
      i *who, what, where, when* questions about all patterns.
      ii beginning of *why* questions
      iii questions about attributes (descriptive language)
      iv use of *do*-support in questions

*As students progress in the simple sentence stage, exposure to complex language should be increased. It is not necessary for a student to master everything in the simple sentence stage before being exposed to complex language.

RECOGNITION

1. Sentence form as meaningful
2. All simple sentence types
3. Question forms
   a) *yes/no* questions
   b) *wh* questions, all types
   c) *did . . . do* questions about verbs
4. Simple adverbs and adjectives
5. General recognition of all pronouns (reference)
6. Prepositional phrases
7. Different forms of negation
8. Infinitive complements
9. Conjunction
   a) in NP_2
   b) simple sentence conjunction
10. Tenses where appropriate
11. Story form
   a) set phrases ("Once upon a time")
   b) anticipatory language (*but . . . so . . .*)
12. Basic conversational skills
   a) when it is time to speak
   b) appropriate social language
   c) appropriate language play and language routines
13. Where there are different languages in home and in school, it is important that the student from the non-English speaking home recognize this difference by the end of this stage.

COMPREHENSION

1. Five basic sentence patterns used in experience stories, social studies lessons, stories, etc.
2. *Yes/no* questions
3. Negatives in simple sentences
4. Simple adverbs and adjectives
5. Prepositional phrases in context
6. Personal pronouns
7. Beginnings of complex language where context is appropriate
   a) infinitive complements
   b) simple, event, conjunction
   c) some causation
   d) adverbial clauses
8. Sentence types
   a) imperatives
   b) interrogatives
   c) declaratives
9. Simple sentence transformations
   a) adverb movement
   b) question formation
   c) *do*-support
   d) negations

PRODUCTION

1. Simple sentences with correct word order
2. Question forms with correct word order
3. Imperatives with correct word order
4. Appropriate intonation with sentence types
5. Basic sequencing relationships
6. Basic conversational skills
7. Different forms of functional language
   a) jokes
   b) riddles
   c) routine greetings

READING

1. Simple sentences
2. Simple sequencing language for plots, adverbials, prepositional phrases, etc.
3. Descriptive language
   a) language marking stereotypical characters (e.g., "wicked witch")
4. Simple read and do exercises
5. Appropriate children's literature
6. Beginning word problems in mathematics
7. Different story forms
   a) plays
   b) short stories
   c) myths and fairy tales
   d) biographies

WRITING

1. Linguistic parameters: In the simple sentence stage, it is hoped that students will attain Level V (Figure 3.9).
2. Compositional Skills: In the simple sentence stage, it is hoped that students will attain Level III (Figure 3.10).

ANALYSIS (formal language skills)

1. Sentence pattern identification, all patterns
2. Analysis by underlining
   a) noun phrases
   b) verbs
   c) adverbials, adjectives, etc.
3. Can identify subject and object noun phrase
4. Possible introduction of tree diagrams where appropriate.

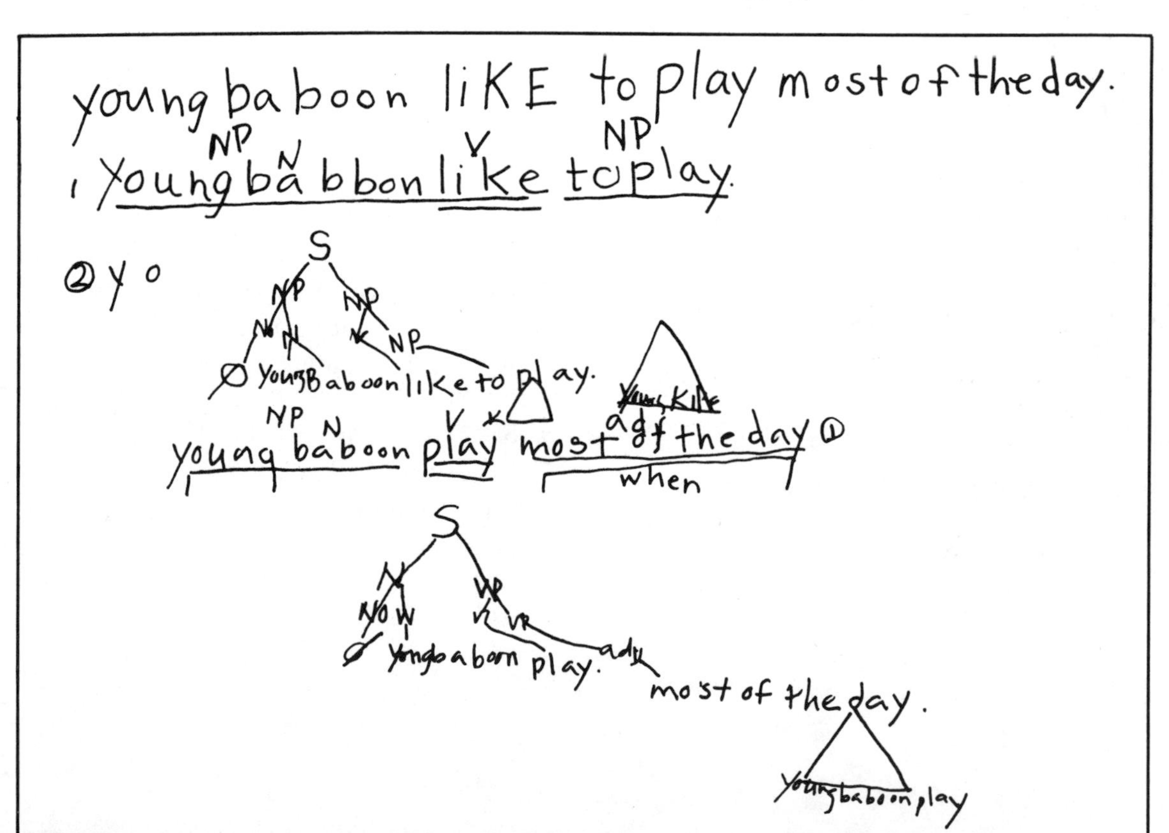

FIGURE 3.15 *Sentence analysis by an 11-year-old student at the Rhode Island School for the Deaf.*

LANGUAGE DEVELOPMENT OUTLINE: Complexity

EXPOSURE

1. Full exposure to all necessary language to describe and sequence experiences.
2. Exposure to structures in contrast
3. Some syntactic considerations
   a) *because* sentences
   b) *if/then* sentences
   c) *There is . . . It is . . .*
   d) relational conjunction
   e) indirect speech
   f) indirect questions
   g) relative clauses
   h) passive voice
   i) pronominalization across sentences
   j) movement of adverbial clauses
4. Dialogue
5. Wide range of affective language
6. Idiomatic usage
7. Organized language play and games (codes, pig-latin)
8. Different languages
9. Projective language

RECOGNITION

1. Syntactic considerations
   a) NP Complements (infinitive, that)
   b) *for* and *by* phrases
   c) prepositional phrases other than directional (*about, of*)
   d) simple sentence transformations
      i passive
      ii dative
      iii adverb movement
      iv question formation
      v various forms of negation
   e) complex sentences
      i *if/then*
      ii *because*
      iii *but, so*
      iv relative clauses
      v multiple embeddings
      vi pronominalization and references across sentences
      vii *where* and *when* clauses
      viii sentence vs. clausal adverbs
      ix embedded questions

COMPREHENSION (follows Recognition very closely at this stage)

1. Question forms
   a) *yes/no*
   b) all *wh*-questions, including *how*
   c) indirect questioning
   d) embedded questions
2. Principles of pronouns and references
3. Movement principles
   a) within sentences (e.g., dative)
   b) with two sentences (e.g., extra-position)
   c) pronominalization across sentences
4. Subordination
   a) relative clauses
5. Conjunction: Movement in this period from comprehension of simple to relational conjunction
6. Descriptive language and its functions
   a) characterization
   b) affective expression
7. Jokes, code play, puns, aphorisms

PRODUCTION

1. Accurate simple sentences
2. Conjoined sentences
3. Conjoined Noun Phrases and Verb Phrases
4. Indirect referencing, using pronominalization
5. Adverbials
6. *Yes/no* questions with use of *do*-support

7. All *wh*-questions
8. Stress and intonation appropriate to the meaning, function and complexity of the sentence
9. Descriptive language
10. Different language functions (jokes, lies, secrets)
11. Appropriate range of affective language

READING

1. Extensive use of children's literature
2. Individualized reading programs
3. Reading each other's writing (for point of view, narrative awareness)
4. Math word problems
5. Advanced social studies materials (e.g., "Man: A Course of Study")
6. Use of fiction with characterization, motive, etc.
7. Use of anticipatory strategies

WRITING (The following sequence might be observable)

1. Simple sentences, all patterns in the beginning of this stage
2. Beginning use of description in beginning of this stage
3. Accurate word order in simple sentences and in early expansions
4. Move to paragraph form in this period
5. Expect more accurate morphology
6. If simple sentences are mastered, expect the student to begin to write complex sentences by the end of this stage
7. Move to more than one paragraph in expansion of complexity

ANALYSIS

1. Kernelization of complex sentences
2. Expanded use of tree diagrams
   a) adverbials
   b) relative clauses
   c) Noun Phrase complements
   d) conjunction
   e) other movement rules
3. Identification of sentence patterns of embedded sentence
4. Underlining identification of *wh* clauses
5. Underlining of *by, for, because* clauses

Chapter 4

The Language Program for Preschool and Kindergarten

Most early childhood or preschool programs begin the formal language education of the hearing-impaired child at around 3 years of age. Generally, the child at this age has had little or no language therapy, has not had or has not learned to utilize amplification and may even have additional handicaps. A consistent language development program and curriculum–one that helps the child acquire language and at the same time allows the teacher to be diagnostic about what is happening in the classroom–will help the teacher more adequately with these problems. Although some fairly specific guidelines will be set for the development of formal language work in the classroom, all the classroom experiences in a preschool or kindergarten should be seen as language experiences.

Early Language Goals

The core of a language program for preschool and kindergarten includes four major goals. The first goal is to provide exposure to the ever-widening experiences and activities which help develop the child's concept of self, how he relates to others and how he relates to his physical environment.

A second goal is to expose the child to the symbolic representation of these experiences in simple sentences. Providing this linguistic information in the preschool is mostly a process of teacher input. The production of these linguistic structures representing experience should be encouraged at a level appropriate to the language development of each child.

A third goal is that the child establishes an awareness or recognition that linguistic representations have predictable structures. A first level of awareness will probably include a sense for word order, the basic Noun Phrase-Verb Phrase relationship, and should lead to a more complex sense of grammar.

A fourth goal of a preschool program is to develop an awareness of the differing forms of language (e.g., rhymes, poems, stories) and an awareness that these forms can serve different functions. The child should recognize that language can represent information; that it can represent immediate experiences as well as events that have not occurred or may never occur (as in fairy tales).

Formal language work is introduced to the preschooler at 4 or 5 years of age. This beginning of formal language work is also the beginning of the process outlined in Chapter 3 by which the enactive and iconic experiences of the child become symbolic experiences as well. Thus, as preschool teachers embark on the task of preparing the best possible environment for language acquisition, they must also be helping the child to go beyond the enactive and iconic processes to a more abstract, symbolic level. At this point it is linguistic representation that is the key form of symbolic representation, especially for the hearing impaired.

The variation in linguistic systems of preschool hearing-impaired children makes it difficult to generalize about where to start and how to begin a language development program. If the child is congenitally severely

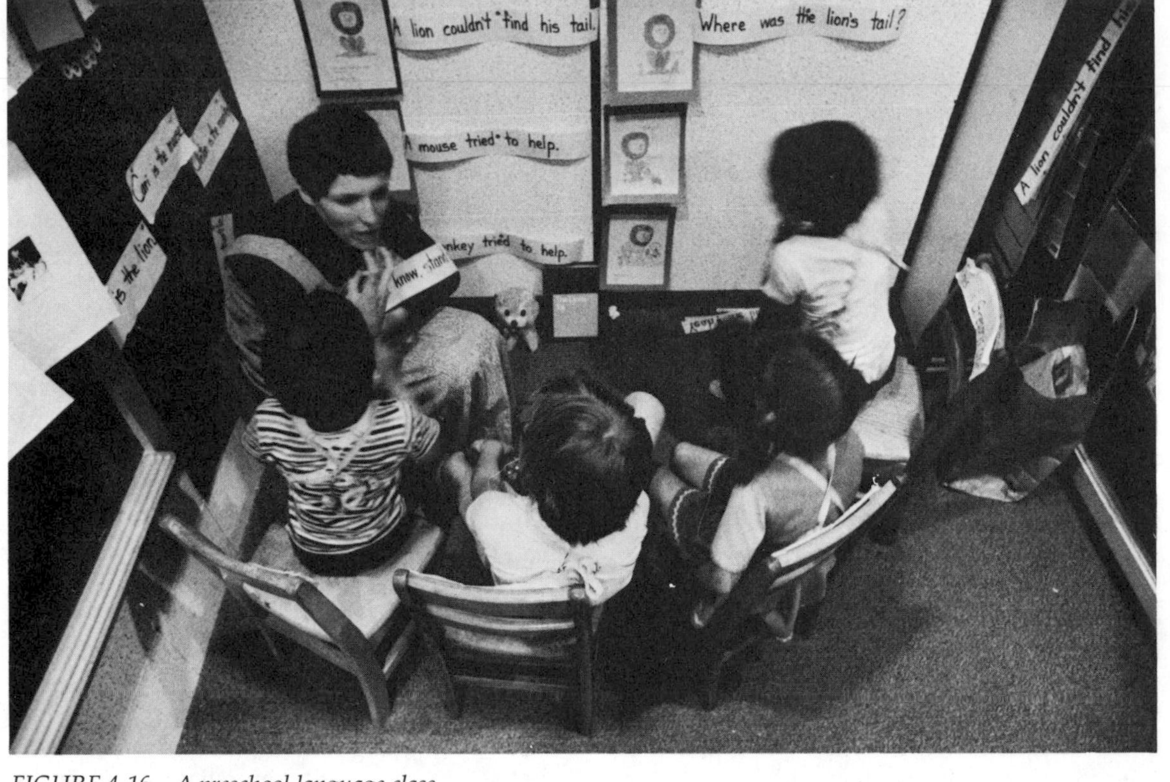
A lion couldn't find his tail.
Where was the lion's tail?
A mouse tried to help.
A lion couldn't find

FIGURE 4.16 A preschool language class

to profoundly deaf, a gesture system or an organized sign language system may be operating. Children with moderate to severe hearing losses may have a fairly well-developed phonological system. For some children, perhaps deafened between one and three years of age, there may be the beginnings of a linguistic system acquired during those early years before becoming deaf. There are, however, some parameters of linguistic form, structure and content that can be discussed as appropriate to most preschool programs for the hearing impaired.

EXPOSURE TO SYMBOLIC REPRESENTATION

For many children, exposure to organized language and thought in school is their first experience with conscious, symbolic organization of the world around them. For many of these children, being asked a question to which a response is required is a relatively infrequent event at home. Due to frequent misunderstandings among parents of hearing-impaired children as to what their child is capable of responding, hearing-impaired children often enter a preschool without ever having had a story read slowly and carefully to them. It is more important for the preschool teacher of the hearing impaired to expose her students to the experiences and language necessary for further linguistic and cognitive growth than to formally teach them anything at this point. The goals of the classroom are to encourage a categorizing process on the part of the child which is more than the mastery of a specific body of knowledge.

Two areas are important in discussing the material that the child is exposed to in preschool: the form and function of the material and the cognitive and linguistic issues considered in relation to this material.

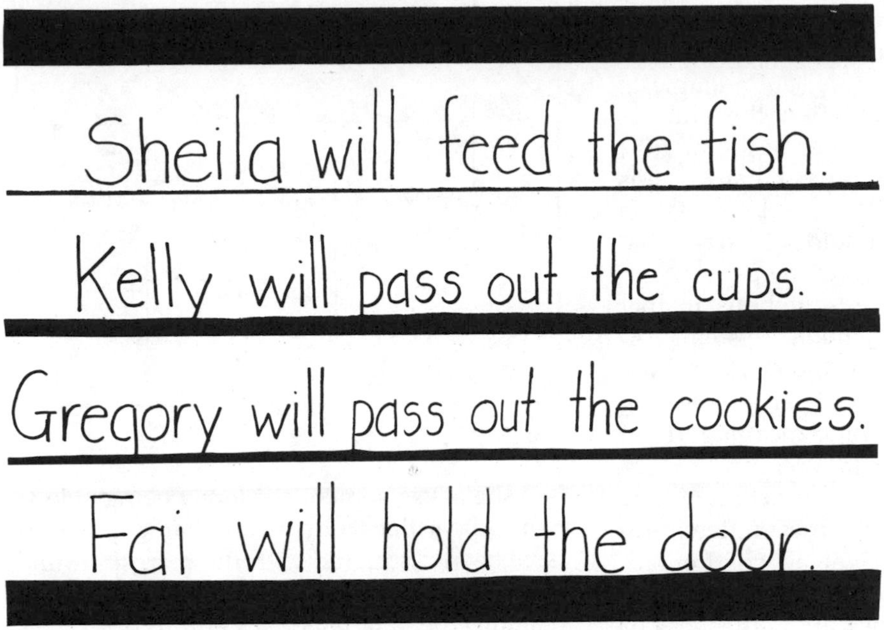

Sheila will feed the fish.

Kelly will pass out the cups.

Gregory will pass out the cookies.

Fai will hold the door.

FIGURE 4.17 Language can function to organize classroom activities

FORM AND FUNCTION OF LANGUAGE IN THE PRESCHOOL

The preschool experience usually begins the first real period of exposure to print for the hearing-impaired child. Depending upon his earlier experiences, the child may have been exposed to verbal language of some kind but probably has had only limited exposure to print: a few greeting cards at Christmas or a children's book or two. But it is at school that the real organizing of print as a form of language is likely to begin. That the print form may be new, confusing or even frightening for the child must be kept in mind. Thus, the well-illustrated experience story written on a chart becomes an important form of written language in the preschool. Songs, rhymes or language games can also be written out on charts and added to the language displayed in the room. *(FIGURE 4.16)* Stories on charts, language lessons, counting games and any and all kinds of classroom language activities should be included in the process of exposure to print.

The various forms of linguistic representations in the classroom are often related to the functions of language. Involving the child in enough situations where language helps to order the world can help him to understand the advantages for learning it.

For example, the early morning assignment of classroom responsibilities can be done with sentence strips. *(FIGURE 4.17)* Not only does this approach lend itself to work on questions and answers, but the child hopefully learns that the written representation also tells who has what jobs and is therefore a source of information also. If a child forgets his or her particular job, the teacher can use these sentences for a lesson on gaining information from printed materials (the informative value of print) rather than lecturing on the importance of paying attention. Integrating language work and classroom procedures is a good way of exposing the child to language in action: functional language.

The child is exposed to many other forms of linguistic representation during this period. Calendars, for example, are a staple of preschool programs but often the child is asked to memorize the names of the months of the year or days of the week before he is even aware that a calendar is a representation of time. The teacher should be aware that calendars, number tables or maps are very much like linguistic representations in that they too are abstract symbolic systems. At this stage, one is exposing the child to those representations and not necessarily expecting the child to understand their meaning. *(FIGURE 4.18)* How well children respond to representation of time is often a function of how well they have established cognitive categories related to time. Not all children respond to the representation of time, particularly with reference to the days of the week or months of the year, in the same way. Children are event oriented at these early stages and utilize these events to organize time.

One hearing child, for instance, went to nursery school on Mondays, Wednesdays and Fridays. She did not know at the beginning which day was Monday, Wednesday or Friday, but she knew that it must be one of those days because she was getting ready for nursery school. The other days were organized according to the events which occurred regularly on each of these days. And, because nothing significant happened on Thursday, the child had difficulty fitting that day into the system and for quite a time functioned without a Thursday. After a period of maturation with questions such as, "What is the name of today?" and later finding something by which to organize Thursday, it was soon a regular part of the system.

Another child the same age did not organize the days of the week quite as analytically. "Sesame Street" and exposure to peers had given her a song which helped her to easily memorize and say the days of the week. The problem was, she did not know whether it was Monday, Tuesday, or any other day un-

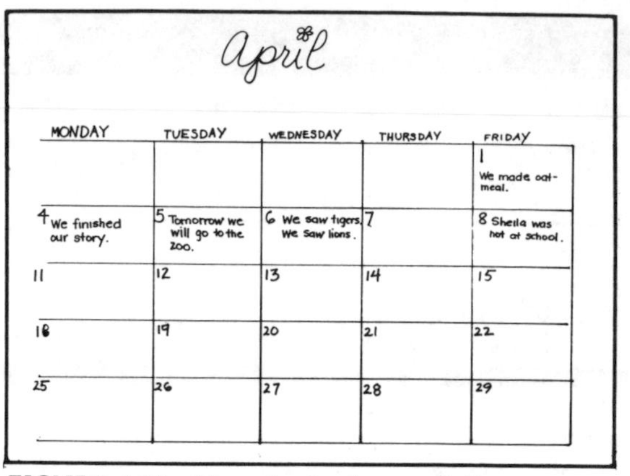

FIGURE 4.18 The calendar is a symbolic representation of school experiences.

less she asked someone. Merely being able to name days does not mean that the names have been associated with the corresponding days. That child needed to find some way of relating the language system to the days themselves.

Likewise, it is not unusual for children to function for quite some time with only two months in the year—December (because it's Christmas!) and their birthday month. The other months are too vague or the time span too great to be of real interest to the very young child.

A mistake parents often make with the young child is to say, "It is five days to your birthday!," only to have the child wake up each morning to ask "Is it five days yet, Mommy?" Out of exasperation, mother resorts to event functioning rather than time measurement and says, "No, it is three more sleeps!" This usually satisfies the child, who is much more comfortable with that kind of organization. The point is, children are not incapable of organizing the days of the week or the months of the year; they may be using a system different from the adult to organize that information, and parents and teachers may spare themselves frustration by being more aware of those systems.

Prime goals of this preschool period are for children to understand that language can represent experience and that using language pays off. In general, then, the language work that a young preschool child is exposed to should be directed at general goals rather than specific informational goals.

One of the language skills that needs to be mastered at this young age is the recognition that there are various functions of language; that is, that language is not doing the same thing on all occasions. Sometimes language gives information, whereas at another time it is for enjoyment only. For instance, in introducing a group of 3-year-old hearing-impaired children to the category of nursery rhymes for the first time, a teacher prepared a series of well-illustrated flash cards for "Three Blind Mice." By the time they got to "She cut off their tails with a carving knife," the looks on the faces of the children ranged from confusion to horror. The teacher realized that there was no reason why the children should not interpret this in the same way as the actual experience of "Trip to the Fire Station" since the language was presented in the same sentence/picture format.

She put away the cards and had the children dramatize the nursery rhyme so that the children became the mice and the farmer's wife. Through this dramatization, the children came to realize that a nursery rhyme was not the same as an experience chart. Exposing the child to the contrast between language for fun and language for information is necessary to arrive at this distinction. In this example, once a category for nursery rhyme was established, it was necessary and easy to enlarge that experience so that the categories of language for experience and nursery rhyme grew in contrast to each other.

There are, of course, other clues which help the child to identify the various forms of language. Fairy tales, for instance, have very recognizable formats that usually begin with "Once upon a time," and end "happily ever after." These opening and closing clues alert the child to the fact that a fairy tale is being read rather than an account of a class field trip, and that one should react with feelings and attitudes appropriate to fairy tales rather than the more realistic expectations of the experience chart.

CONTENT OF THE LANGUAGE PROGRAM

The content organization underlying language at the preschool level revolves around several basic notions:

1) Content work, at the earliest levels, is conceptually based and is aimed at establishing a network of inferences. Patience in giving adequate, meaningful exposure is necessary but the teacher should not prematurely expect conceptual recognition as well.

2) Language is the representation of a conceptual framework and therefore, if conceptual recognition happens, then language can happen. The opposite is not necessarily true; language structures to which the child does not bring conceptual organization may not be meaningful.

3) The ability to recognize and understand language, both at early and later stages, will be greater than the ability to produce language. Therefore, production should be measured as a process in and of itself, and accepted as only a minimal measure of the comprehension abilities of the child. The exposure to language should be at a level that is not just a reflection of what the child can produce, but also reflects the teacher's intuitions about the conceptual and linguistic recognition abilities of the child.

"The Three Bears," the first story in one reading series, contains the familiar lines:

> Papa Bear's porridge was too hot.
> Mamma Bear's porridge was too cold.
> Baby Bear's porridge was just right.

The final sentence contains the phrase *just right* in contrast to the earlier *too hot* and *too cold*. To comprehend the story, the child must be able to contrast things being *too hot* or *too cold*, and the problem's solution of *just right*. Hearing children may bring mature concepts to the story and therefore have no trouble

We made oatmeal.
We poured oatmeal into the bowl.
John poured cold water into
the bowl.
Sally stirred the oatmeal.
Everyone tasted the oatmeal.
It tasted awful!
Yuck!
It was too cold.

FIGURE 4.19

understanding it as is. Hearing-impaired children, however, may need help in establishing such conceptual relationships.

It is not unusual for preschool programs to include projects such as making jello or popcorn. Why not oatmeal (to be later called porridge)? One teacher involved the class in making oatmeal with cold water. In tasting it the class made it very obvious what they thought of cold oatmeal. This can be written, then, as an experience chart. *(FIGURE 4.19)*

Several days later the experience was repeated, this time using boiling hot water. One child was courageous enough to try to taste it, but that was all as the message was made abundantly clear that it was too hot! The child's production, at this time, may only be the word *hot*, which is usually one of the first words produced by hearing children. A similar chart is written and recognition of some structures should occur. *(FIGURE 4.20)*

By the time the children read "The Three Bears," the concepts of too hot and too cold (especially on the part of Joseph) had been learned and the process moved quickly from recognition of a similar experience and structure to comprehension of the story's events.

The preschool program, in this limited set of lessons, contained a balance of personal experience and story material and utilized a good set of sentences that could become part

We made oatmeal.
We poured it into the bowl.
Mrs. Smith poured hot water
into the bowl.
Sally stirred the oatmeal.
Joseph tasted it.
He burned his tongue.
The oatmeal was too hot.
We waited.
It was just right.

FIGURE 4.20

of formal language work. These sentences can be used for recognition work, such as matching or discrimination activities, as well as speech for auditory training.

As children become more comfortable with print and are able to recognize some of the sentences used in the experience of making oatmeal, the teacher may begin writing some of the familiar sentences on large oaktag charts. Two charts might initially be entitled SENTENCES and used for grouping sentences according to their syntax, though no formal reference is made to the structures involved. *(FIGURE 4.21)*

Sentences from succeeding stories or events may be added to these charts and used in exercises matching picture to sentence and sentence with sentence, and in identifying a particular sentence in response to the request "Show me . . . ."

There is now available in the classroom a collection of familiar sentences with contrasting syntactic structures. When it comes time to talk about syntax, these sentences are an invaluable set of shared experiences in sentence form.

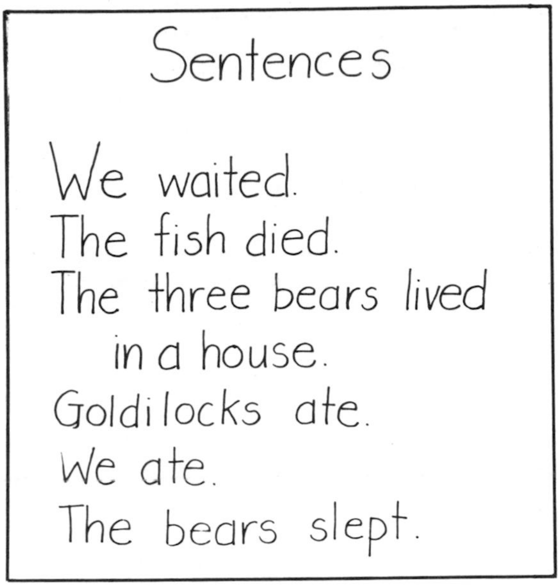

Sentences

We waited.
The fish died.
The three bears lived
in a house.
Goldilocks ate.
We ate.
The bears slept.

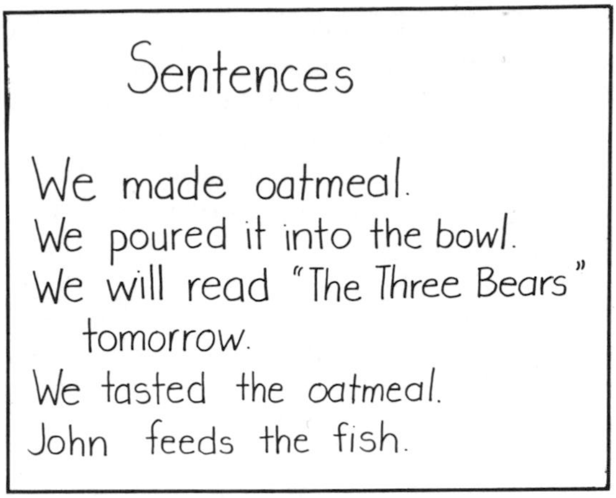

Sentences

We made oatmeal.
We poured it into the bowl.
We will read "The Three Bears"
tomorrow.
We tasted the oatmeal.
John feeds the fish.

FIGURE 4.21

Pronouns

Questions raised by teachers regarding the sentences listed on the charts or used in the various lessons often relate to what pronouns should be introduced. A very common approach to pronoun work in schools is to change proper names in a sentence, usually gained from a news lesson, to pronouns.

John watched TV last night.
He watched TV last night.

If the experience described by the language is meaningful, there is no reason for children not to acquire pronouns in the same way that they acquire proper names. It may be that there has been too much emphasis on the pronoun/proper noun relationship in the teaching process.

It is also important to evaluate the usual approach of doing pronoun work primarily in subject position. Slobin (1973) points out, however, that hearing children seem to acquire the object pronoun first for two reasons:

1) Object pronouns are usually stressed more than subject pronouns and therefore children attend to them first. Examples of such stress are easily illustrated in games, such as rolling a ball with instructions—"Give it to *him!*" "Roll it to *her!*" "Send it to *me!*"

2) The object pronoun is the dominant syntactic form. Out of eight forms of pronoun usage, object pronouns occur seven times. Consequently, children will overuse object pronouns in sentences such as "*Her* hit me!" and "*Me* want that!" but not so with subject pronouns.

The problem of teaching the verb tenses in preschool language work can be approached in the same manner as pronouns. If the variety of verb tenses used in sentences are presented in contrast, distinctions between past, present and future structures can, for the most part, be learned along the way.

Negatives

Unavoidably with the use of negatives comes the use of *do*, often a trouble spot for language teachers. Action questions in even the simplest pattern one sentence involve the use of two related transformational rules, one called do-support and the other called negative placement.

Pattern one sentence: Sheila jumped.
Question: What did Sheila do?

This *did . . . do* combination may be used by the teacher and even understood by the child, although the child usually uses a negative without do-support in producing sentences such as "I not want that!"

Because this kind of production is very common, it should be noted that the problem is not that a sense for the negative is lacking, but rather a lack in the mastery of the do-support rule. The child may comprehend the question but have difficulties in producing a well-ordered syntactic response.

A dramatization of "The Little Red Hen" might be useful to encourage fluency in the use of negatives and do-support. Little Red Hen asks, "Who wants to help me grind this wheat?"

> "*I don't!*" said the Cat.
> "*I don't!*" said the Dog.
> "*I don't!*" said the Pig.
> "I will do it myself then," said the Little Red Hen.

Studies (Quigley et al., 1976) confirm teachers' observations regarding the tremendous problems experienced by hearing-impaired students with questions containing the do-support rule. Avoidance of these questions will not solve the problem but only perpetuate the children's insecurity with the structure, particularly as it is a common structure in basal readers. While it is not until the next stage of syntactic development that students can be expected to actually comprehend this kind of verb-phrase question, there is little chance of such comprehension if no exposure is given to such questions in the first stage of the program.

These general considerations do not clearly describe the range of language to which the child is exposed. Rather, they point out some areas that must be presented and given attention in the early stages. Many teachers intuitively hit these language spots, knowing the necessity of such exposure.

A Language Development Framework

RECOGNITION/COMPREHENSION

The steps of recognition and comprehension are treated together at this level for one basic reason; most of the language recognized is language understood. Recognition, the awareness of language as language, is a large step for some preschoolers. Having rarely been exposed to an organized or adequate linguistic environment, they can perhaps recognize, understand and use only a few of the functions of language and the forms in which they appear.

Preschoolers might recognize a rise in intonation functioning as a request for something (accompanied by a pointing gesture) or a short vocal outburst indicating no! They may comprehend a particular question, such as "What is your name?", but in general they do not recognize the category of sentences that request information. If children are to make real progress in language development, the recognition of the various forms and functions of language will and must begin to move ahead of actual comprehension.

Toward the end of a preschool program, recognition will move significantly ahead of comprehension for some students but not for others. That is, some children will recognize that they are being asked a question, and may even recognize that the answer is on the chart they have been working on, but might not comprehend the question well enough to answer it. Other students, however, might not recognize the question form at all as a request for information.

Students' inability stems from a different, more pervasive problem at the recognition level. This difference can be used diagnostically, for a student who does not recognize the general forms and functions of linguistic acts is a student who perhaps has not developed an awareness of sentence types or categories of language functions.

Among the most important goals for recognition and comprehension are those relating to the linguistic notion of **sentence types.** Functionally, this is the ability to recognize the difference between a question, a statement, and a command. Linguistically, it is the difference, both syntactically and semantically, between the interrogative, declarative and imperative.

Recognition and comprehension of sentence types and their roles in communication help to establish speaker-receiver relationships and conversational behavior, the cornerstones of linguistic development. This recognition and comprehension of sentence types is an issue independent of mode; those programs that stress heavy aural approaches achieve recognition and comprehension solely through developing the child's use of intonational patterns, while other programs might use a manual system that appropriately (to its own internal structure) indicates sentence types. Whatever the approach, the role of sentence-type differentiation in further language development is crucial and a prime recognition/comprehension goal for a preschool program.

Language plays an important role in organizing the classroom but only insofar as the students recognize that language functions to do that organizing. Seen as part of the acquisition of sentence types, recognition and comprehension of classroom directions are well-conceived and are part of the traditional language goals.

The understanding of particular classroom directions does not happen in isolation from more general language processes. While the language structures used in the directions might vary in terms of syntactic and semantic considerations and goals, the form of the directions is important in itself. After all, there is no reason to expect a 5-year-old child to know, a priori, that just because something is written on a wall in red letters it is an important instruction. The child who pulls the fire alarm might be more than just mischievous; he may not recognize the color or form of the representation which tells him not to touch, even if the words ("Do not activate except in emergency!") are too hard to read. One might teach children the items that should and should not be touched, but more useful is an approach that teaches them to recognize and process the linguistic and paralinguistic cues that convey this information.

Thus, the traditional language objective, "The student will understand classroom directions," involves much more. There is, first of all, the sentence-type distinction. Are all directions imperatives? Is there variation in the syntax, morphology, and lexicon of the directions? Does the child recognize the form and, further, comprehend the content? Can the child use those directions productively? For example, can they "play teacher?" While many children enter a preschool program with virtually no organized system of linguistic representation and with an extremely limited lexicon (regardless of modes of communication), it is expected that by the end of preschool they will not only have the beginnings of an organized system of syntax and semantics, but a receptive competence that enables them to differentiate functional sentence types.

PRODUCTION

The actual production and performance of language by the hearing-impaired preschooler will probably lag far behind his receptive language competence at this point. It is important, then, to look in a positive way at what is produced for what it indicates about the child's language development. That is, by evaluating even the most minimal output in terms of what it indicates about the child's language level and progress rather than by the extent of language delay it indicates, an appropriate language program can be better designed.

In terms of some overall language goals, a major priority is that the child develops an awareness of language as a means of communication in the functional sense; that the child relates whatever systems—oral, manual, written—to each other and to the functions of language. In more specific terms, this means the child should be producing some form of questions, commands and statements. This does not necessarily mean there will be interrogative word order or appropriate morphology, but only that there will be a clear indication in the child's production that this sentence type distinction is present. Intonation patterns might also be clearer in the expression of yes-no questions, even when accompanied by a general interrogative gesture. Interrogative word order in English is, of course, fairly complex and involves several simple sentence transformations.

In general, the production as well as the recognition/comprehension of differentiated forms for different sentence types is a major goal of a preschool language program. In many ways this is an issue independent of content, but in some very basic ways content is very much a part of language structure. Above all, an important part of the preschool curriculum should be one that requires the child to ask questions. The process of language acquisition is an active one, and the child will not learn question structures unless motivated to ask questions.

A child might leave the preschool period with the ability to answer *who* and *what* questions relating to classroom language activities. Answers will be short sentences—two or three words—but in terms of the child's spontaneous productions one would expect fairly well-organized, three-to-five word sentences. "Fairly well organized" is difficult to describe, but the following transcriptions provide some clues in analyzing the productions of preschoolers. (*FIGURE 4.22*)

I forgot
Not now
Push back
Father no work finish
My father finish
Debra cry outside
Boy bad
Debra play
Wash
Miss Evelyn far away
Lisa eat
Lisa paint
Before paint remember?
Boot before remember?
Tomorrow birthday father
Can't hear you

FIGURE 4.22 Partial transcription of spontaneous language of a preschool student at the Rhode Island School for the Deaf. This language sample indicates the establishment of basic word order and semantic relationships.

READING/PRINT RECOGNITION

One of the major differences between the education of a hearing-impaired child and that of the hearing child is that the hearing-impaired child begins reading acquisition at almost the same time as he begins formal progress in language acquisition. The hearing child enters school at about 5 years of age with complex syntax, an almost fully developed phonology and a semantic component that has been shaped and reshaped by continuous feedback from intelligible productions. Few hearing-impaired children come to school with such a full language base.

Presented with a large amount of print for the first time, the hearing child at least has a well-developed language base to bring to this new language form. But the hearing-impaired preschooler begins to read at the same time he or she begins acquiring simple

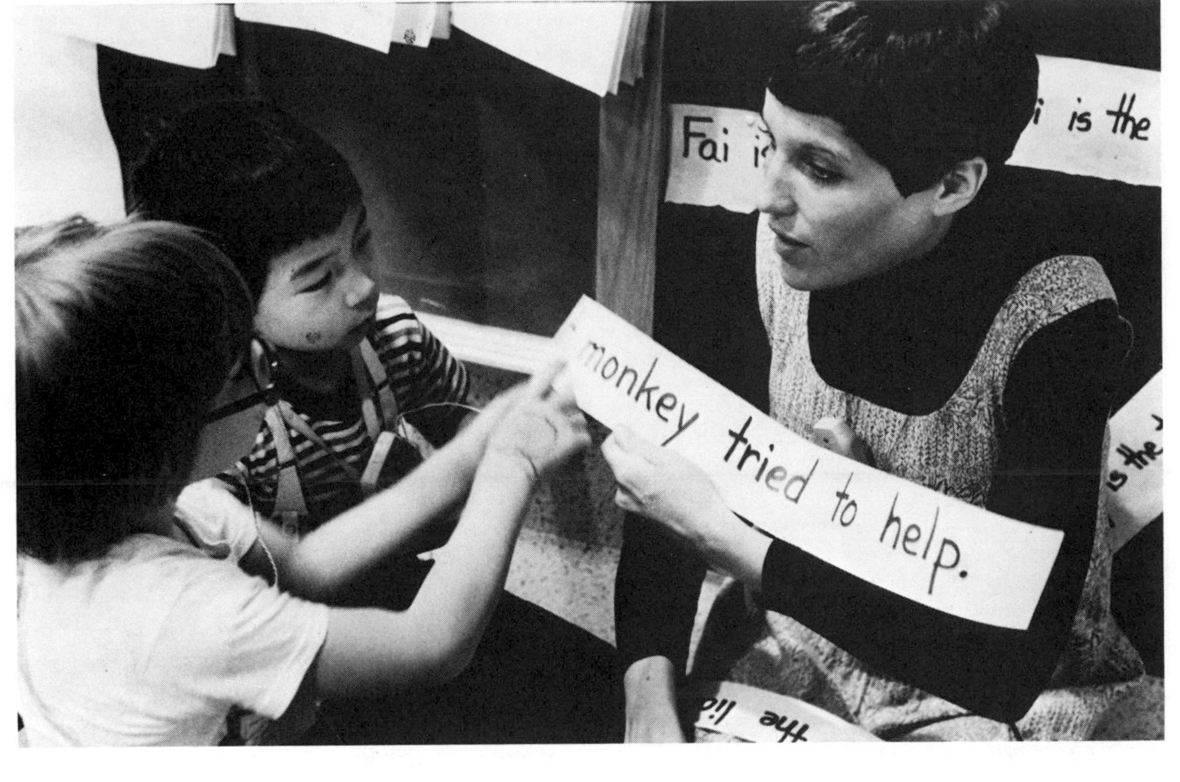

FIGURE 4.23

sentence syntax and producing sentences that make only the most elementary semantic relationships clear. In addition, development of phonology is very delayed and in most cases has resulted in severe speech problems.

Rather than lamenting the need to begin reading instruction when there is little or no established language base as a serious problem, it can be turned into an advantage. That is, the reading component of the language development program is not approached as adjacent to or growing out of language acquisition in general, but as a positive aid in lessening the language problem.

It cannot be assumed in this early exposure to print that the child has an established awareness of grapho-phonemic relationships (letter/sound correspondences) or an awareness of the English alphabet code. It is probable that the child has linked the print next to a picture in some way to the meaning of that picture, but that print is not yet an autonomous, symbolic unit which can stand apart from either the action performed or the pictographic representation. *(FIGURE 4.24)* This whole presentation of picture and print is what the child sees, not the print as another way to represent what has happened. It is quite probable that the print, in this case, is a part of the whole frame or landscape of picture and action. At this stage, the print could not be presented in isolation to represent or signify the event. The first awareness of print as being a signifier perhaps comes with name recognition and the barest minimum of sight vocabulary; i.e., teacher's name, "cat," "dog," "boy," "girl," or with word signifiers like "McDonald's," "Cheerios", etc.

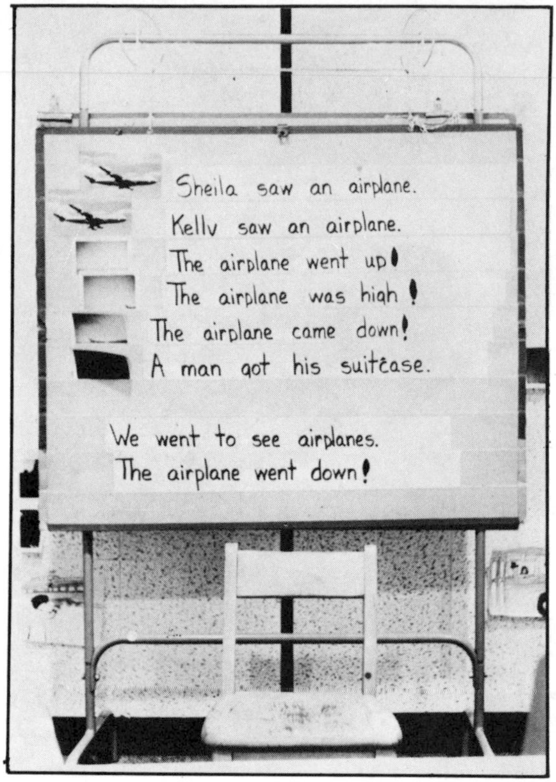

FIGURE 4.24 Early language lessons may involve the presentation of sentences with pictures, but preschoolers often interpret these iconically.

The hearing child in this early language stage functions with an awareness of print as representative of something, and while he may not connect the print to particular linguistic levels, he does know that it means something. Of course, there are some 5-year-old children who do not recognize the word as a unit of anything, but they are the exception. Furthermore, it is very common to see young hearing children having extreme difficulty breaking words down into letters, identifying words with similar sounds, or even blending phonemes to form words. Despite these difficulties, many hearing children still recognize that graphic forms are a code for spoken language.

What can be achieved in preschool is creating a disposition in the child to accept written language and reading as highly communicative, enjoyable and informative experiences. Good stories presented over and over again are one way to ensure this.

Experience stories, rhymes and tales can be made into an illustrated book form. The print on the pages can be one or two sentences repeated intermittently throughout the text. *(FIGURE 4.25)* This is reminiscent of the primers of the 1940s and 1950s and, although some educators have criticized this format, the target of their complaints–the repetition and monotony–may be what helps the young hearing-impaired child to read.

A child needs some kind of assurance that the page can be dealt with independently. On one level, there are the pictures; on another level, letters may provide some cue that helps him decode meaning. On still another level, the child may realize a pattern of repetition where he does not even have to read the second word carefully to get the meaning. These basic awarenesses should be given a chance to work as the young reader is exposed to more and more meaningful print.

It is hoped that the awareness of printed material as a **code,** that is, a symbol that signifies or represents something else, can be reached by the time children enter lower school. Such awareness expands the teacher's ability to capitalize on the students' reading readiness skills.

Reading seen as a perceptual skill requires selection and combination of stimuli. Like most learned behaviors, it depends on concepts and skills learned previously. Many of them, for the hearing-impaired child, are not specifically picked up before entering school.

Aside from language, there is also a wealth of visual and auditory stimuli which surround the child. The biggest problem lies in what kinds of "chunks" children organize their perceptual experiences. Adult "chunking" of perceptions is based on a more sophisticated system than a child's, but children also see patterns and use them as functional categories.

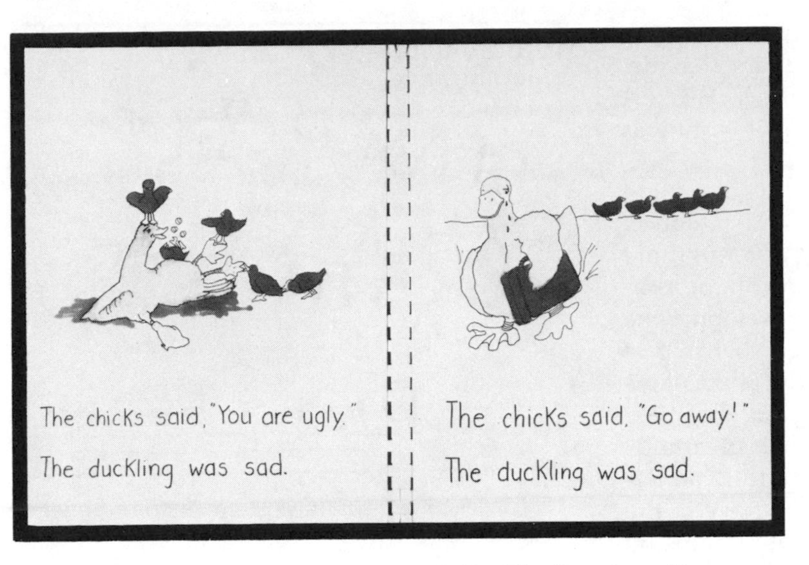
The chicks said, "You are ugly."
The duckling was sad.
The chicks said, "Go away!"
The duckling was sad.

FIGURE 4.25 The popular tale "The Ugly Duckling" can be written using a simple repetitive format in a hand-made book.

Attending to and identifying distinctive features of both auditory and visual stimuli are things that cannot be put aside until children are actually trying to read printed sentences from charts and books. The auditory patterns of rhythm and intonation are one kind of perceptual chunking that prereaders and early readers can learn to use and rely on in reading.

Although reading readiness training will not be discussed here (the literature is more than adequate in this field), research has shown that a very important factor in the later success of readers is caused by the early exposure to letters and configuration (Gibson & Levin, 1975). Prereading children do not know much about letter sequencing in their language code, but they can manipulate the distinctive features which make up the forms of that code. Auditory and visual gaming and copying can play an important part in helping to prepare for reading performance. A memory component should be built into these activities as well. The goal, at this point, is to make the visual and auditory stimuli as familiar as possible, and to encourage the child to categorize these stimuli.

WRITING IN THE PRESCHOOL

As was pointed out in the section on reading in the preschool, most hearing-impaired children's exposure to written language occurs simultaneously with their first processes of language acquisition. The same seems to apply to writing; that is, preschool children start to manipulate letters, scribble, copy their names and perform other writing tasks at about the same time that they are first really beginning to acquire language in an organized way. Because of this sudden confrontation with language in different forms, special care must be taken with writing as well as with reading to see that both processes are carefully integrated into the overall language program.

Several considerations of what must precede real productive and information-carrying writing are necessary in the preschool. First, there must be a way of developing recognition of writing as a communicative process. For example, each child might have a personal mailbox in the preschool area and this might be used to receive mail. Even though the children are scribbling or only rotely copying their names onto scraps of paper, these might become letters that the students can send to one another. This is just one way of attempting to establish writing as a form of communication.

Encouraging the mechanical act of writing is also a consideration in the preschool. Firstly, this establishes writing as a fun thing to do and one that pays off in communication. Scribbling is also part of developing the eye-hand-language coordination that is part of writing. If the child readily begins this scribbling-as-expression process, the next move is to a level of identification of sounds and letters. This may begin with the first letter of the child's name and then move to the identification of another classmate's name by first letter. This is often associated with some form of written language play and, like other forms of language play, is to be encouraged.

One hearing child, for example, found a small notebook which looked similar to the order pads that waiters and waitresses use. She immediately became a waitress and asked,

> "What do you want to eat, Dad?" Father replied, "I'll have a hamburger."
> "What else?"
> "Some french fries and a coke, please."
> "What do you want for desert?"
> "Some pie."

The resulting list on the little pad was *FIGURE 4.26* The spelling and vocabulary were not an issue here, but it was the joy of the role playing and the significant role of writing in that act that was the focus for the child. These activities can be promoted in preschool by having writing materials readily available, by establishing a writing time and area for students and by each child having his own personalized writing book or journal.

Many schools for the hearing impaired also have in their population children with learning disabilities in addition to hearing loss. In some cases, physical problems created by the disease that deafened the child (cerebral palsy, meningitis) also make the writing process difficult. The high percentage of hearing-impaired students with visual problems is also a concern here. For these children, the actual physical process of drawing letters on paper might be difficult. But this does not mean they cannot "write." Use of cut-out or plastic, three-dimensional letters is a possibility for children who have trouble holding a pencil, and success with these letters might provide the motivation for learning how to write with a pencil.

These individual letters are not only important for multiply handicapped children but for other children as well. For example, in the Rhode Island preschool there is an area of the room that has a large cabinet covered with magnetic letters. The children spontaneously play with this array frequently and hardly a day passes where there is not a name or word spelled anew amongst the letters.

By the end of preschool it is hoped that students are comfortable with writing as a means of communication, are actively scribbling and playing with the written form and are trying to express meaning in their writing. Until enough linguistic structure, even at the phoneme/grapheme correspondence level, is present, it is difficult to assess the child's meaning or attempts to express meaning.

Writing with a purpose . . .

HMBRG
KOK
FANTHEIS
PI

FIGURE 4.26 The function of early writing can be simply the act of writing itself.

But it must be remembered that the child who is actively writing, even if that writing is unintelligible scribbling, thinks that he or she is saying something. It is a common experience for children to come up to their teachers and provide a long interpretation of one scribbled word. Moreover, they are often shocked when the teacher does not immediately understand the meaning of what they have written. One child in the Rhode Island School for the Deaf handed her teacher a collection of word-like assemblages of letters which she described as a list of people in her class. When asked where her teacher's name was, the child showed her a seemingly jumbled series of letters. Although the teacher could not actually read her name, this code approximation was meaningful and functional for the child.

Above all, writing in the preschool should be an enjoyable experience for the child. There should be ample opportunity for child-dominated writing activities in self-expression, as well as a balance of copying of names and early sentences and other teacher-dominated activities that provide some necessary structure to the writing process. Teachers should be aware of a developing linguistic level in any writing; beginning phoneme/grapheme correspondences or even the grouping of scribbles or letters by word type groups. Function is another consideration and the child should particularly be exposed to the communicative functions of writing.

If student and teacher view writing as only a burdensome part of the day devoted to penmanship practice, independent of context and experience, language development is not enhanced. Integrated into the overall curriculum, writing becomes useful, fun and communicative and this is a positive factor in a child's overall language development.

ACKNOWLEDGMENTS

FIGURES

Page 54 *Figure 4.16* Photograph courtesy of Ira Garber

Page 55 *Figure 4.17* From unit prepared by Judy Tartaglia, Rhode Island School for the Deaf.

Page 56 *Figure 4.18,* Page 58 *Figure 4.20,* Page 59 *Figure 4.21,* From unit prepared by Joanne McCaulley, Rhode Island School for the Deaf.

Page 63 *Figure 4.23* Photograph courtesy of Ira Garber.

Page 64 *Figure 4.24,* Page 65 *Figure 4.25* From unit prepared by Judy Tartaglia, Rhode Island School for the Deaf.

SUGGESTED READINGS

EARLY CHILDHOOD EDUCATION

Bronferbrenner, U. *Two worlds of childhood: U.S.A. and U.S.S.R.* New York: Russell Sage Foundation, 1970.

Caplan, F., & Caplan, T. *The power of play.* New York: Doubleday & Co., 1974.

Cazden, C. Some implications of research on language development for preschool education. In R. Hess & R. Bear (Eds.), *Early education,* Chicago: Aldine, 1968.

Weber, L. *The English infant school and informal education.* Englewood Cliffs, N.J.: Prentice Hall, 1971.

Chapter 5

The Simple Sentence Level

The building of a simple sentence grammar is crucial in the language development of the hearing-impaired child. It is the basis upon which all subsequent development will take place. The child who has difficulty with or is delayed at the simple sentence stage of language acquisition will soon fall behind in other related areas, such as reading, understanding the content material of the lower and middle school curricula, and developing written language. More importantly the child will not have the language structures needed to express his growing cognitive skills.

As noted earlier, a language curriculum should present linguistic data to the child in a form that will help him acquire the linguistic rules of his language. This is especially important at the stage where acquisition of a hierarchical system of language structure begins and an awareness of the predictable and stable structuring of sentences develops.

One way of presenting useful linguistic data at this level is by utilizing the basic sentence patterns of English. These linguistic structures express the simple grammatical relationships of the language, the **kernel sentences,** which serve as the language building blocks for the simple sentence stage. They are not goals in and of themselves but only ways of organizing the basic linguistic structures to be mastered during beginning stages of development.

The sentence pattern approach is an outgrowth of structural linguistics and also of the earliest theories of transformational grammar. In those early formulations (Chomsky, 1957; Harris, 1964 [in Fodor & Katz, 1965]), the grammar was conceived as a system where the phrase-structure rules generated kernel sentences, and the transformational component of the grammar acted on those kernels.

". . . the grammar of a language can be hierarchized into an elementary part, called the 'kernel' of the language, and a second part which consists of a set of transformational rules for deriving complex sentences from simple ones. The kernel grammar contains the definitions of the main parts of speech and describes rules for constructing simple declarative statements without complex noun and verb phrases. The transformational rules then carry these kernel sentences into other sentences or into phrase or clause segments of sentences, which could not be derived in the kernel grammar" (Braine, 1967, [in Jakobovits & Miron, 1969, p. 249]).

Two concepts growing out of the kernel sentence approach serve as a starting place in the presentation of language. The first concept is that **big sentences are made up of little sentences** and the second, that big meanings are made of little meanings. Our objective then is to help the child acquire those little (simple) sentences needed to develop the big (complex) sentences.

Even in the first Rhode Island Language Curriculum there was an awareness of some problems with the kernel sentence theory. According to Blackwell and Hamel (1971):

"Although we recognize that the concept of kernel sentences has been de-emphasized in later linguistic material, we feel it is a helpful basis for a language program for deaf children" (p. 57).

While the curriculum has seen many changes corresponding to advances in linguistics, the usefulness of the kernel sentence approach in a language program for hearing-impaired children remains.

The Five Basic Sentence Patterns As Illustrated in the 1971 Rhode Island School for the Deaf Language Curriculum

	Labels	Sentence
Pattern 1	who	The baby cries.
Pattern 2	who, what	The baby drinks milk.
Pattern 3	who, adj.	The baby is cute.
Pattern 4	who, who	The baby is a boy.
Pattern 5	who, where	The baby is in the crib.

Source: *Rhode Island School for the Deaf Language Curriculum,* 1971, p. 62.

The Five Basic Sentence Patterns As Currently Represented at the Rhode Island School for the Deaf

	Sentence	Labels
Pattern 1:	The baby cries.	NP V
Pattern 2:	The baby drinks milk.	NP_1 V NP_2
Pattern 3:	The baby is cute.	NP LV Adjective
Pattern 4:	The baby is a boy.	NP LV NP
Pattern 5:	The baby is in the crib.	NP LV Adverbial

FIGURE 5.27 The five basic sentence patterns

There are several major differences between the use of the five basic sentence patterns in the 1971 Language Curriculum and in the current curriculum. It might therefore be helpful to briefly discuss the theoretical and methodological issues in the sentence pattern approach.

The interrelatedness of the patterns is a major point of emphasis that did not appear in the 1971 Language Curriculum. This is illustrated by the interdependence of the development of one pattern on the development of others and the resulting classroom strategy of presenting patterns in contrast. Interestingly, it was the importance of the contrast principle in the acquisition of complex sentences that led to consideration of the role of contrast in simple sentence structures. Patterns are no longer taught one by one, with mastery of one pattern a prerequisite for exposure to the next one.

The second major difference is the emphasis on semantic relationships in simple sentences and particularly the role of the verb and verb phrase in the acquisition of sentence structure. *(FIGURE 5.27)*

As presented in the 1971 Curriculum, there is an emphasis on classification by *who* and *what, where* and *when.* The animate/inanimate distinction in the noun phrase seems to have been the only important distinction in the lower school program. The adjective is a grammatical category stranded in pattern three, and the contrast between expanded pattern one and pattern five, as well as other contrasts between and within basic patterns, are not marked in the older notation. According to the new curriculum, semantic differences, as seen when contrasting *how* and *where* questions in both patterns one and five, are now included in the formal presentation of language in lower school.

However, there is danger that the sentence pattern approach will be interpreted as a circumscribed and controlled approach to language presentation; that it will be used in a rigid, nongenerative way. This approach is not meant to be utilized as a slot-filling system. These are not patterns into which one mechanically drops "parts of speech." Rather, these structures express the basic grammatical relationships of our language - relationships the child must acquire in order to understand and be understood.

As an example, many (but not all) of the world's languages are subject-verb-object

(S-V-O) languages. English is a language of this type. To express the meaning that somebody did something to somebody else a structure is needed with just that word order. Pattern two presents this S-V-O relationship in its noun phrase-verb phrase-noun phrase (NP-VP-NP) structure. Anyone who has had experience with young, hearing-impaired children knows the frustration of not understanding the message the child is trying to express when this crucial word order has not yet been acquired.

One of Lois Bloom's contributions to the field of child language was her observation that children acquiring English use word order meaningfully as soon as they begin to produce two-word utterances. As she says, "*the consistency with which the surface order corresponded to the inherent grammatical relation within the utterance was impressive*" (Bloom, 1973, p. 11).

Roger Brown (1973), in discussing Bloom's argument for the evidence of word order, elaborates further:

"*With two words, two orders are possible, with three words, six orders. The child's use of just that order which is appropriate in the model language for the relations existing in the situation, an order corresponding to the inclination of the interpreting adult, constitutes a kind of discriminating response on the child's part giving evidence that he and not only the observing adult has certain semantic relations in mind* (p. 148).

The acquisition of word order, as a means of expressing semantic relations and as a means of giving the child a way to express what he knows about the world, is one of the objectives in presenting language in sentence patterns. In the beginning, therefore, the content of the sentence patterns should be optimally meaningful. That is, the sentences should express something the child has experienced, already "knows," or is in the process of learning. The use of a sentence pattern out of context, or one that is unrelated to the child's experience, will not help him to connect this linguistic representation to something that he understands conceptually. In initial exposure to new patterns, old information should be used. Later the contrast between old and new information can be highlighted through the use of familiar patterns.

The long term goal, of course, is for the child to internalize linguistic structures so they can be used spontaneously and meaningfully. The child should eventually understand that the grammatical relationships expressed by the NP-VP-NP order (pattern two) are the same, even if the ideas and specific vocabulary used are unfamiliar. The child must acquire the ability to identify who or what is acting, what the action is, and who or what is being acted upon in any pattern two sentence. This is the essence of acquisition of linguistic structure.

These considerations motivated the change from the oversimplified schema of the 1971 Curriculum to the present edition, although the basic validity of the five basic patterns remains. An awareness of the use of the patterns, of how they relate and how they express meaning, makes the patterns more meaningful. In essence, present understanding of the patterns has changed, but not the sentence patterns themselves. Seen in this new light, patterns remain a useful tool in designing a language development program for hearing-impaired students.

The Five Basic Sentence Patterns

SENTENCE PATTERN ONE

The first sentence pattern consists of a noun phrase and a verb phrase:

The baby cries
NP VP

As simple as this sentence is, it contains the basis for the first phrase structure rule of a transformational grammar:

S → NP + VP

The child will probably master this pattern by the end of the preschool program. Mastery at this point is not judged by analysis skills but by general productivity of the pattern, comprehension of sentence strips used to describe classroom experiences and the teacher's assessment of whether the child has established a consistent system for differentiating between names (NPs) and actions (VPs). This latter point, the differentiation between NPs and VPs and not the ability to mechanically segment two- and three-word sentences, is the motivation behind sentence pattern one and a goal of the language work on this pattern.

Sentence pattern one is often varied by the addition of an adverbial.

1. The owl hoots at night.
2. Yesterday, the class played.
3. Kelly laughed loudly.
4. John went home.

In sentence 1, *at night* is a prepositional phrase functioning as an adverbial answering the question *when*. In sentence 2, *yesterday* functions in the same way but its position in the sentence is different. The contrast between adverbials in initial position and final position is one that students must acquire to become successful manipulators of language.

Sentence 3 is also different for it has a manner adverbial, *loudly*. *Loudly* answers a *how* question as contrasted to the *when* question *(at night)*. The morphological marking, the *-ly*, is a surface structure clue that signals semantic differences. While it is necessary for students to make efficient use of surface structure clues, it is the deep structure relationships and the semantic contrasts signaled by the morphology that must be acquired.

In sentence 4 a noun is functioning as an adverbial. If the sentence patterns are only used as a slot-filler grammar, where parts of speech are dropped into structural slots, this appears to be a pattern two. But the semantic function of *home* is adverbial and this deep structure difference is what must be understood by both student and teacher. Establishing these semantic contrasts within pattern one is important for further syntactic development because other syntactic processes and distinctions rest upon these earlier ones.

For example, the difference between patterns one and two depends upon one of the contrasts outlined within pattern one.

5. John went home. (pattern one)
6. John likes his home. (pattern two)

Processing these two sentences requires the student to understand that a given lexical item, in this case *home*, can function as an adverbial (answering a *where* question) or as an object noun phrase (answering a *what* question). Unless the student recognizes the underlying linguistic structure (the deep structure), the morphological information provided by the possessive pronoun *(his)* is of little or no use in processing these sentences.

If the student is comfortable with the range of contrasts within sentence pattern one, the contrast between patterns one and two is easier to establish. Exposure to different types of pattern one sentences and pattern two sentences begins early and, although the basic form of the pattern may have been mastered in preschool, final mastery of this semantic difference might not come until later in the simple sentence stage. Since adverbials within pattern one sentences concern relationships of space and time, the child's cognitive development and the growth of a semantic system are closely related to the acquisition of the linguistic structures that express these relationships.

SENTENCE PATTERN TWO

The boy	hit	the ball.
NP_1	V	NP_2

Pattern two expresses the Actor-Action-Object semantic relationship in English and is one of the earliest and most frequently acquired basic sentence patterns for any child.

In the 1971 Curriculum, much attention was given to which verbs were really pattern two and which verbs were not, and much of this discussion was centered around the role of the passive transformation and the transitive/intransitive distinction. These questions have not disappeared but the answers no longer concern attempts to list verbs by predetermined categories. Instead, the function and meaning of the whole sentence is considered. This important feature was reaffirmed by the statement in the 1971 Curriculum that *"the five patterns used in this Curriculum indicate basic sentence types according to their kernel phrase structure rather than on the basis of verb or word type or of exceptions in the application of transformational rules"* (p. 60). While there is some reemphasis on the role of the verb in the revised curriculum, it is the semantic interpretation and syntactic functioning of verbs in the context of sentences that is important.

The current use of sentence pattern two by lower school teachers at the Rhode Island School for the Deaf concentrates on several areas not mentioned in the 1971 Curriculum and deemphasizes some of the more structural aspects of the earlier formulation. Among the new areas are: the contrasting of pattern two with other patterns,the difficulty of questions asked about the verb in pattern two (the *did . . . do* construction) and the importance of what can appear in the NP_2 constituent (e.g., infinitive, compound NP). Deemphasized is the attention given to the animate/inanimate classification of nouns as seen in the *who/what* distinction. An increased awareness of the semantic function of pattern two, the carrying of the Actor-Action-Object meaning, is superimposed above syntactic considerations, especially in the use of this pattern in the classroom.

SENTENCE PATTERN THREE

The sun feels warm.

The	building	is	tall
	NP	be/LV	Adj.

Sentence pattern three is the first of the patterns using linking verbs such as *tastes, feels, seems.* It is also the first pattern that involves the verb *to be* and, not surprisingly, pattern three is reported to be the most difficult to teach by those who have been using the Rhode Island sentence pattern approach over the last few years. Since patterns four and five also involve the verb *to be* and the linking verbs, the probable explanation for both teacher and student difficulty with pattern three may be the occurrence of the category adjective. In patterns four and five, NPs or adverbials follow the *be*/linking verb, but in pattern three it is the adjective that follows. The students have had success with NPs and adverbials following the verb in patterns one and two and thus patterns four and five are identified by their contrasting verb types and meanings.

Yet pattern three is approached with little previous syntactic or semantic representation to provide direct contrast of structures. In addition, productive use of adjectives is often indicative of a child who uses attributes to categorize experience. Too often the hearing-impaired child between 6 and 9 years of age is still functioning on the event level. Thus, patterns two and five, which sequence events, might seem easier to teach at this stage.

The difficulty with pattern three only serves to reemphasize its importance. At the simple sentence stage, mastery of this pattern might prove difficult. But it is important that the child be exposed to a wide variety of descriptive language so that, as classification by attribute becomes important, the linguistic tools that support this cognitive development are available.

Sentence pattern three is also important because of its contrasts with pattern two. As Blackwell and Hamel (1971) note: *"As many of the linking verbs are related to the senses, feel, taste, smell, etc., there may be a linking verb in Pattern Three but a transitive verb in Pattern Two when used with a predicate NP (e.g., Larry tasted the soup* [*pattern two*]. *The soup tasted lousy* [*pattern three*])" (p.62).

As shown earlier, this syntactic contrast also brings out a semantic contrast; new and old information as they are used in contrasting sentences. In the first sentence *the soup* is the new information (assuming Larry is a member of the class). Moving to subject position, *soup* becomes old information for the student. This makes the concentration on an attribute of the soup much easier. This kind of language exercise not only takes advantage of the functions of subject position in sentences but provides valuable contrast between patterns two and three.

A further step with this contrast might be the use of pronouns in these patterns:

Next, Billy tasted the soup.
It tasted lousy.

If the student knows the lexical item *soup* and understands the structure, there is no need to "explain" the pronoun, *it*. Contrasting patterns is not only important for the contrast itself but it also increases flexibility for both teacher and student in language work. The contrasting of syntactic patterns through the use of the new information/old information contrast should be an ever present consideration in preparing language materials or lessons.

SENTENCE PATTERN FOUR

The student	became	a teacher.
NP	be LV	NP

Sentence pattern four also employs the so-called *be*/linking verb, but again it emphasizes the semantic nature of the verb. As noted in the 1971 Curriculum, the verbs used in pattern four are semantically verbs of process or the verb *to be*.

The man	was	a baker.
NP_1		NP_2

Notice that in this sentence the noun phrases are identical in reference. While the noun phrases are different words and differ in meaning, they refer to the same original object. Pattern four, then, is the basic linguistic form for representing one thing changing into another but still related to its previous self. As in pattern three, thinking by attribute as well as conservation of various attributes are involved in pattern four. The two sentences,

The beanstalk became a tower.
The beanstalk became scary.

illustrate that a child must recognize the contrasting syntactic structures as well as understand the process of change to make semantic sense of the sentences.

SENTENCE PATTERN FIVE

Monkeys	are	in the jungle.
NP	be/LV	Adv.

My house	is	on the hill.
NP	be LV	Adv.

Sentence pattern five is described very succinctly in the 1971 Language Curriculum,

Sentence Pattern Five occurs less frequently than any other sentence pattern and is the structure NP-LV (be only)-Adverb (where, when) (p. 62).

Examples are as follows:

The ball is on the table.
The game was on Tuesday.
He is outside.

After several years of working with this minimal syntactic description, the semantic import of this pattern and its relationship to other patterns became clearer: pattern five contrasts with patterns one and three. While the child is working on the adverbial expansion of pattern one, pattern five might also be used contrastively.

The children played in the gym (pattern one).
The children are in the gym (pattern five).

Many teachers using the Rhode Island approach over the last few years have worked on patterns four and five before three. It may be that the student's experience with the verb *to be* in pattern five paves the way for mastery of pattern three. Cognitively, pattern five depends upon conceptions of space and time, which ideally the child is developing during this simple sentence stage.

Using the Sentence Patterns in the Classroom

Keeping the goals of the previous section in mind, it might be helpful at this point to describe some ways in which sentence patterns can be used in the classroom.

The first step is to work through the sentences with the class to ensure that the concepts are understood and the vocabulary is familiar. It is particularly important in the initial work on language structure that progress not be hampered by unfamiliar vocabulary and that the child understands a small set of vocabulary to use in presenting sentence patterns. However, this does **not** mean that a list of vocabulary is first taught in isolation.

It is also important at this stage that the sentences are understood conceptually and that the children are comfortable with the methods used in presenting language in sentence patterns. At about 7 years of age, the child should be able to move into sentence analysis as a part of formal language work. *(FIGURE 5.28)* It should be emphasized again that this method or technique is merely one of many tools that will help children look at language they understand conceptually from a strictly linguistic point of view. Students are asked here to develop their metalinguistic abilities; that is, to use language to talk about language as a way of developing a sense of syntax. This development of increased metalinguistic awareness is felt to be an important and positive factor in the overall acquisition and development of language.

The use of sentence analysis helps the child develop the categorical concepts that make up a well-formed sentence; that is, noun phrases, verb phrases, adjectives and adverbials. This initial step will eventually lead to an understanding of the function of these categories and their relationship to each other. While some labeling is part of the teaching process, it is the understanding of the underlying relationship rather than the surface labeling that is the goal of sentence analysis.

There are several ways to approach the labeling of categories. Some teachers use *who, what, where* for instance, as the first labeling of sentence parts. Others may begin with such labels as Noun Phrase or Verb Phrase. The important consideration is not what kind of labels are used, but that the labeling is meaningful to the child and will lead to productive, useful categories. The use of sentence analysis, as the use of sentence patterns, is not an end in itself but simply a step along the way toward the development of complexity. When the child reaches the level of complex sentences, his ability to analyze sentences to determine what kernels are present will be a very useful tool.

One of the important aspects of acquiring a grammar is the ability to know what goes with what in a sentence, or put more formally, the ability to phrase or to identify the constituents of a sentence. The child must reach a point where he understands that, in spite of the varying lengths and complexity, a group of sentences are made up of similar constituents.

Sentence analysis can also help the hearing-impaired child identify the auditory chunks that he is unable to fully hear. Sentences that are understood and have been analyzed by the child can be creatively used in speech work to develop a sense of phrasing, sentence contour and intonation.

SENTENCE ANALYSIS

As mentioned in Chapter 4, sentences that represent a variety of experiences have been classified for some time on oak tag charts according to their syntactic structure or sentence pattern. As a result, when analysis or description of the grammar is introduced formally, a selection of familiar sentences of each type is available on the oak tag charts.

In the description of these sentences, the appropriate use of the question transformation can help to identify the relationship between the constituents within a sentence and prevent the rote labeling of vocabulary items according to a predetermined part of speech. For instance in the following sentences,

1. We went to Florida last winter.
2. Last winter was cold.

the traditional identification of *last winter* as *when* works quite well in the identification of that constituent in sentence 1. But in sentence 2, *last winter* does not answer *when*.

By applying the appropriate questions to these sentences, the appropriate semantic function of the constituent is identified.

1. We went to Florida last winter.

Q. When did we go to Florida?

A. We went to Florida *last winter*. (when)

2. Last winter was cold.

Q. What was cold?

A. *Last winter* was cold. (what)

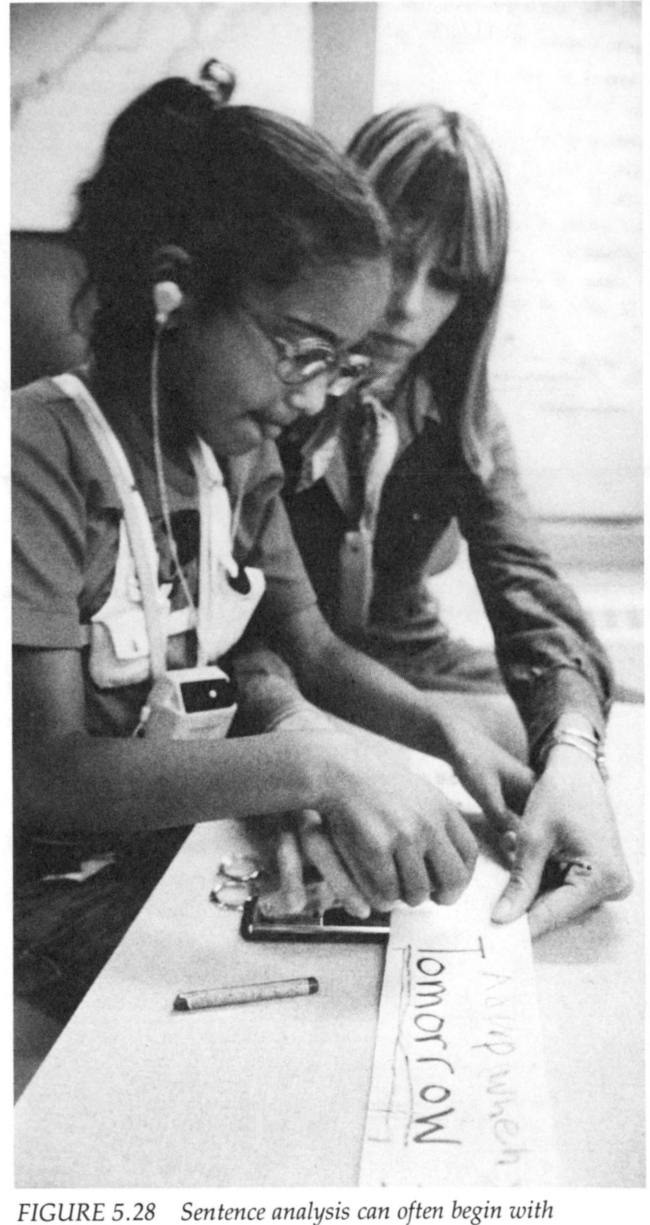

FIGURE 5.28 Sentence analysis can often begin with sentence strips that can be cut up, moved and labeled.

SENTENCE ANALYSIS PROCEDURES

The format for introducing analysis might be:

1. Introduce sentences describing concepts in a unit.

   We see many insects around us.

2. Select sentences from units and other activities and list according to syntactic structure or sentence pattern. No formal reference needs to be made to sentence pattern formulas.

   A spider crawls.
   A bee flies.
   A bee builds hives.
   A spider weaves a web.
   A spider is an insect.
   A bee is an insect.

3. (A) Choose a sentence from the chart for discussion and write it on the blackboard or overhead.

   A spider crawls.

   (B) Have the child read the sentence. Check for comprehension.

   "Show me the spider."
   Child points to illustration on chart.

   (C) Question the Subject Noun Phrase (NP).

   Q: "What crawls?"
   A: A spider crawls.

   (D) Identify spider as either *what* or Noun Phrase

   A spider (what) crawls. or A spider (NP) crawls.

   (E) Choose another sentence for Subject NP identification.

   A bee (what) flies. or A bee (NP) flies.

4. When children are spontaneously answering questions about Subject NPs, identify Verb or Verb Phrase (VP). Some teachers have found that identifying the verb by labeling it is sufficient. Others prefer to question the VP.

   Q: "What does a spider do?"
   or Q: "What did Ann do?"

We see many insects around us. A spider is an insect. A spider crawls. He weaves a web. A spider catches other insects in his web.

A bee is an insect. He flies. A bee builds a hive. The hive is his house. The bee makes honey in his hive.

Ann saw a big bee.

Ann ran fast.

5. Utilize similar formats for sentence pattern two, asking questions of the Object NP.

   Q: "What did Ann see?"
   A: Ann saw a big bee (what).
   or Ann saw a big bee (NP).

6. Contrast sentence patterns one and two, giving formulas for both patterns.

   Pattern 1: A spider (NP) crawls (V).
   Pattern 2: A spider (NP_1) weaves (V) a web (NP_2).

   (Anywhere up to a year could be spent on the first pattern until the children are comfortable with the process of analysis.)

7. Continue analysis of sentence patterns three, four, and contrasting verb types *be* with other verb types in sentence patterns one and two only.

   Pattern 1: A caterpillar crawls.
   Pattern 3: A caterpillar is small.
   or
   Pattern 2: A caterpillar spins a cocoon.
   Pattern 4: A caterpillar is an insect.

FIGURE 5.29 Sentence analysis procedures

SIMPLE SENTENCE TRANSFORMATIONS

One thing to be avoided in sentence analysis is the possibility of it becoming a rote function for the child. The separation of sentences into constituents, whether by linear analysis or by "treeing," is a process that the child should think through. That is, the child should be struggling to develop and apply linguistic competence through analysis, not performing a mechanical, memorized sequence of actions.

One way of avoiding this rote performance is to use sentences that are meaningful to the child. These might come from social studies work, stories or often from the student's own productions. If the goal is to relate signal and meaning, having a student analyze a sentence that he or his classmate has spontaneously and meaningfully produced is one way to approach this goal. Analysis makes the student aware that by structuring his signal, his meaning will be clearer. Meaningfulness and context are important parts of comprehending and producing linguistic structures. Language used for analysis must also be presented meaningfully and in context if the analysis is to support the comprehension/production process.

Another way of preventing rote responses is to continually vary the form of the sentences presented for analysis. The child should gradually be acquiring the ability to process longer noun phrases and verb phrases as well as adjusting to variation of position within a phrase. Variation in length and form of sentences, even in the early part of the simple sentence stage, is a way of preventing the student from developing an analytical strategy that always interprets the first word of a phrase as a determiner, the second as a noun, the third as a verb and so on.

Adverb Movement

One of the first transformations used to vary the language presented in the classroom is the adverb movement transformation. It is also related to the development of the expanded sentence pattern one and to sentence pattern five. In pattern one sentences we often use adverbs:

We sang yesterday.

If these adverbs modify the entire sentence, they then can be moved to the front of the sentence:

Yesterday, we sang.

If the adverb only modifies the verb (that is, it is in the verb phrase constituent), then it doesn't sound like a natural sentence of English. (The asterisk in front of a sentence indicates that the sentence is ungrammatical.)

*Fast we ran.

Sentence pattern five also has adverbials, often prepositional phrases that do not move:

The book is on the table.
*On the table the book is.

In sentence pattern two it is often important to add an adverb even though the basic sentence pattern does not mark a space for it:

Yesterday we read a story.
NP_1 V NP_2

This expands the base component of the child's grammar and at the same time allows for transformational variation in the sentence. For the child not to become locked into a rote strategy of analysis and to have the data for generalizations as to which adverbs can be moved and which cannot, this variation of simple sentences should be utilized. In addition, when the child moves into complex sentences he will be able to apply the principles arrived at for movement of simple adverbs to the movement of adverbial clauses.

Simple sentence transformations participate in the changing of form and meaning in sentences that contain only one verb phrase. According to earlier theories of transformational-generative grammar (T-G), transformations did not change meaning (Chomsky, 1957). But later views of T-G accepted that transformations, like the negative transformation, do in fact take part in the changing of meaning in a sentence. Even though the negative may be generated in the base component of a grammar, it is the transformation that converts this underlying negation to a surface negative sentence. Thus, when a student is asked to change a positive sentence into a negative sentence, the student must use syntactic rules that make changes in meaning expressible. In the same way, a transformation such as do-support is mostly a grammatical support operation, while a transformation like question formation not only involves a change of meaning, but a change of sentence type as well as representing an important linguistic function. While transformations like dative movement (Mary gave the book *to me.* → Mary gave *me* the book.), and particle movement (John put *on* his coat. → John put his coat *on*.) seem to be simply optional word orderings, the passive (*John* hit Mary. → *Mary* was hit *by John.*) is a transformation that depends on stylistic choice and on semantic notions of topic and comment.

Teachers should understand that not all transformations carry the same weight in importance and function. Transformations are represented in formal grammars by the same notational system and format, but transformations do not all have the same functions. The question transformation is a vital tool for the language teacher and is used constantly in class, while the passive might seldom appear. Although both are simple sentence transformations, a child who cannot form questions is in far worse shape, linguistically speaking, than the child who cannot quite decipher the passive. A child who cannot adequately formulate negatives is far more likely to be misunderstood or to misunderstand than the child whose particle movement rule is not sensitive to the occurrence of a pronoun. In order for the child to escape the generalization that all transformations are the same, teachers might avoid presenting them mechanically without regard to their function, importance or meaning. As in the use of analysis in general, the occurrence of simple sentence transformations in a language lesson or program is not a random sprinkling of structures and transformations but should depend on the meaningfulness, form and function of that particular transformation and its appropriateness to the language being presented.

A hearing child brings to the learning process, particularly reading and writing, an internalized language base that includes many of the preceding structures. The hearing-impaired student, however, is confronted with particle movement, dative, passive and other forms in readers and books, while at the same time acquiring the rules of a simple grammar.

It seems advantageous, then, for the teacher to not only be aware of the comprehension and productive language functioning of the child, but also to be cognizant of linguistic forms as they appear in classroom material and to use them, on one hand, to facilitate language learning, and on the other, to enable the children to respond appropriately to the material.

Reading and Literature in the Simple Sentence Stage

One could write volumes on the hows of the reading process and the methods of reading instruction. Judging from the debates about which approaches are most effective–look say or phonics, structured or natural language, basal readers or children's literature–the volumes would somewhat resemble the chronicles of the British Wars. Mere surface knowledge of the controversies, both theoretical and practical, will indicate that no one approach to reading instruction produces what Sloan (1975) calls *"literate readers, those who not only know how to read, but who read fluently, responsively and because they want to"* (p. 1).

Although the emphasis in early reading is conventionally on teaching reading skills (those which allow the reader to respond automatically to the written word), active reading ability must also be developed. No matter what the approach, it is finally the task of the teacher to set down her own signature on the reading program which evolves.

Much of the literature on beginning reading instruction deals with those reading skills commonly identified as "word attack" or "phonics." These skills, however, will be discussed only so far as they apply in developing reading programs for the hearing impaired. The conventional methods of phonics instruction are based on rules of phoneme-to-grapheme (or sound-to-letter) correspondence. The discussion of phonics will also include those regular spelling patterns that yield common visual configurations in written language. Although word recognition cannot simply be defined in terms of visual-auditory discriminations, a great deal of early reading requires that perceptual information be extracted, combined or associated.

The reading process is most immediately facilitated or hindered by the structures used by the reader to order the textual information before him. Structures, in this context, are organizing units that define the many levels on which reading occurs: the phonemic, syntactic and extended discourse levels. **Phonemic structures** are internally regularized spelling patterns as well as letter-sound correspondences. Structures on the **syntactic level** permit the reader to use the constraints and redundancies of language. Structures on the **extended discourse** (prose) level allow for inferential readings. *"The reader processes the largest structural unit that he is capable of perceiving and that is adaptive (has utility) for the task he is engaged in"* (Gibson & Levin, 1975, p. 294). The reading performance goes quickly beyond the text-dependent processes of decoding or translating, and even beyond psycholinguistic guessing (Goodman, 1967). The linguistic information alone cannot tell the reader about actions, their consequences and their effect on people. These things have to be inferred from the text; if not, the passage will remain a serial account. Miller (1965) points out that the meaning an utterance may carry is not the linear sum of the meanings of the words that compose it. A meaningful understanding of E. Dickinson's statement, "A word is dead . . ." or Dylan Thomas' "a grief ago . ." is not the sum of its parts.

Weiner and Cromer (1967) defined reading as a distinctive type of thinking in which the assimilation of meaning is a function of both the thoughts and words of the writer and the extrapolation processes of the reader. These extrapolation processes demand creativity as well as reading skill. The readers' judgments of his own performance, as well as his expectations for the printed page, constantly redefine reading, the reader, and the text. Effective readers think effectively. Teachers of the hearing impaired realize the importance of reading for thought as well as for improving and practicing communication skills.

If one is to comprehend a word, a phrase, a sentence or a text, both the linguistic information within the text and the extratextual information which the reader himself brings to the reading task are necessary. Carroll (1972) distinguished "pure" comprehension of this linguistic data (straight language comprehension) from other, more sophisticated kinds of comprehension which make inferences and deductions that go beyond the text itself.

The reader, then, must actively perform while reading. For example, when one picks up a box of Jello and begins reading the directions, or when one opens "Snow White" to the first page, an active response is demanded. With recipes, the function of reading is to bake or cook something and the reader's performance will be overt: mixing, combining, measuring. However, active reading can also be covert. A young reader beginning "Snow White" actively performs by anticipating the huntsman's slaying of "Snow White." It is important to promote reading that actively engages the reader, the text and the writer.

Just as our students cannot be taught all the words or sentences they will need, teachers cannot possibly find and then teach all the reading materials they will need. Instead, teachers can give students as many skills as possible to deal with the materials and choose materials that develop the abilities that make good readers.

EARLY READING AND THE HEARING IMPAIRED

As the child leaves preschool, the demands made on his language and reading behavior change greatly. The prereader approaches the early elementary grades having been exposed to many simple sentence patterns in varied enactive contexts, as well as with a minimal sight vocabulary which relies on initial letters, features of length and general configurations. However, this awareness of sentence types and highly frequent sight words will not necessarily allow the child to read within the next one or two years. Nonetheless, the written language he is presented with, whether experience-based or story-based, requires the lower school child to recognize many new words, to structure these words into larger units or phrases, and to comprehend what he has read. This process of learning to read will be rewarding if the child is given as many useful strategies for decoding as possible and if the written material with which he is presented is manageable as well as meaningful.

The reading strategies accessible to the elementary school reader will depend on those emphasized by the program's approach to reading. Some may build a reading curriculum around the language structures being taught, others around phonic analysis of new vocabulary, and still others around sight words whose meanings are to come from use of contextual and extratextual constraints. The child in a structured language program may therefore be more predisposed to use a known language pattern than context clues to recognize or guess the meaning of a new sentence. If oral modeling is used to teach reading, then the child will most likely work with the sound-letter code and will "sound-out." A vocabulary-oriented approach may lead the child to depend on word meanings and the associational relationships as derived from the child's experience.

The approach to beginning reading most often discussed is that which emphasizes the code. Some research suggests (Chall, 1967) that for normal children, programs which initially emphasize cracking the alphabet code (mapping sound to symbol) produce better readers by the fourth grade. The problems of these readers are less serious than those in programs that begin teaching reading with attention to meaning.

Still other researchers argue for a meaning-emphasis approach where children learn to decode written information using an understanding of the message rather than the code. Meaning is derived from context clues, vocabulary knowledge and reader involvement with the content.

Both of these approaches and their varied methodological manifestations assume that the child comes to school with an adequate receptive and expressive language base. This is not true for hearing-impaired children. In the lower school experience where many of the language structures to be acquired are presented in written form, reading performance is not easily distinguished from language learning. While language functioning is clearly part of reading performance, reading performance for the hearing-impaired child may often influence the language learning process itself. The unanswered question, then, is if teachers are asking for reading on both the graphic-decoding level and the syntactic-semantic level, how and when do these two processing levels interact, facilitate

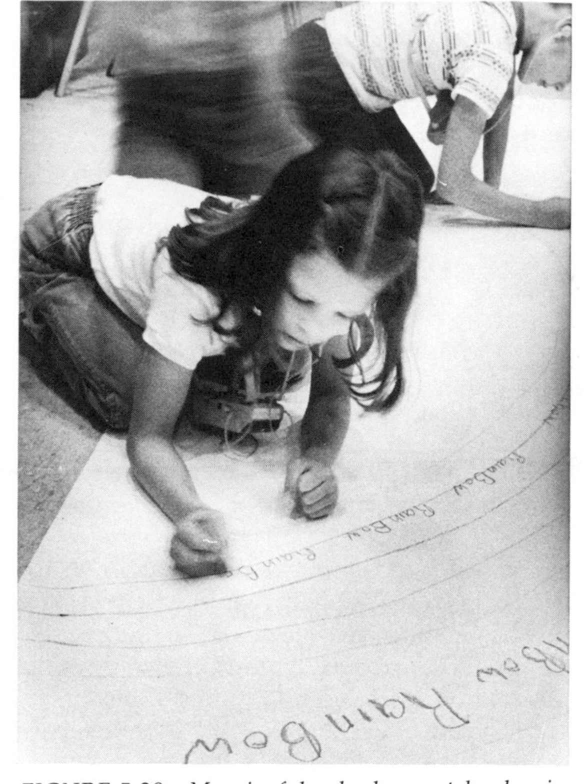

FIGURE 5.30 *Meaningful code play can take place in the art room as well as during language arts.*

each other, or possibly interfere with each other? A diagnostic issue which faces the lower school teacher as a result of this question is what a reading-decoding problem is as opposed to a reading-language problem.

Just as there are times during a language analysis lesson when the child may not go beyond surface structure manipulation of the pattern, so are there times in reading when the child may not go beyond simple code play. The teacher can recognize and encourage the reader who, in manipulating words, discovers that the word *stone* also contains the meaningful segment *one*. The teacher should extend this spontaneously initiated code play by constructing reading activities in class which relate this play to meaningful decoding skills. *(FIGURE 5.30)*

Another curriculum issue which must be confronted by the lower school teacher is the

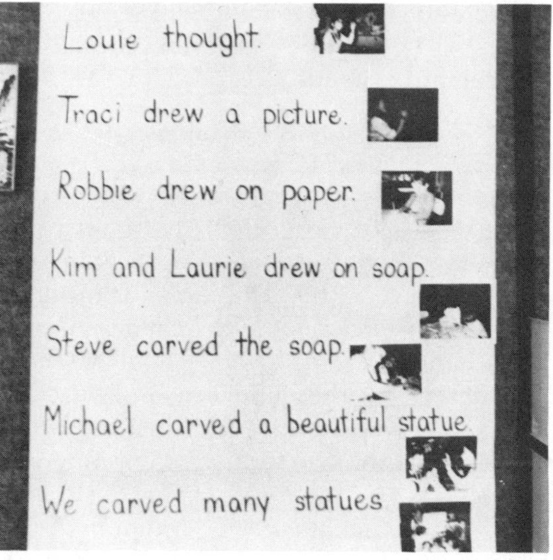
Louie thought.
Traci drew a picture.
Robbie drew on paper.
Kim and Laurie drew on soap.
Steve carved the soap.
Michael carved a beautiful statue.
We carved many statues

FIGURE 5.31 *The linguistic representation in chart form of a first year lower school experience.*

dependency of reading skills upon language skills. The widely used language experience approach attempts to minimize this dependence by prefacing actual reading with group activities. It is hoped that the commonality of experience will carry enough meaningful clues for the beginning reader to understand the written representation without relying exclusively on reading, decoding or language skills. *(FIGURE 5.31)* But, because reading materials such as fairy tales, fantasies and adventures soon move away from the enactive immediacy of experience, skills that help the child use the actual printed material must, at the very least, be made available in the early school years.

"The great debate" over whether to emphasize reading as decoding or reading as deriving meaning (Chall, 1967) may be inappropriate, then, for the hearing-impaired child. The hearing child's language and experience base precedes his confronting the reading code and perhaps a phonic emphasis which highlights and objectifies the nature of the code is needed early or from the start. For the hearing-impaired reader, however, the emphasis is often reversed. A conceptual base is established early and the specific phonic and linguistic skills which help him understand what he reads are introduced as the program expands.

LOWER SCHOOL CHART FORMS

As noted earlier, a problem of which to be aware in designing written classroom material is that both language and reading are being learned at the same time. The organized language behavior of the child in his first and second years of lower school has been fully described; the child can recognize the basic sentence patterns and is just beginning to use them to structure his own language productions. If this development is to continue, the readability of the written materials that present these and more advanced structures is a serious consideration.

The chart story is a very important part of the lower school experience. In the early grades, the chart form is used to present in printed (or symbolic) form the enactive experiences that everyone has participated in. There is much discussion of events and each student's unique perception of the experience is included in the chart. *(FIGURE 5.32)* The chart form is also suitable for stories adapted from classics, fairy tales and children's literature (i.e., Hansel and Gretel or Midsummer Night's Dream). The informative content of social studies and science units can also be written in chart form.

For young readers, the task of reading in the sense of giving an overt response to a particular text is, at first, a form of paired-associate learning; each written word is matched to either a signed and/or spoken response. This associative stage (Samuels, 1970) in which the child reads word by word without necessarily understanding these words is a natural and universal one and should be seen as part of the process of learning to read. The child's ability to go beyond the word, an ability especially easy to overestimate in the hearing-impaired child who depends heavily on extratextual clues, is necessary if the child is to make use of larger structural units while actually reading the text. It is the design of chart stories which, through careful construction, should help develop this and other important reading skills.

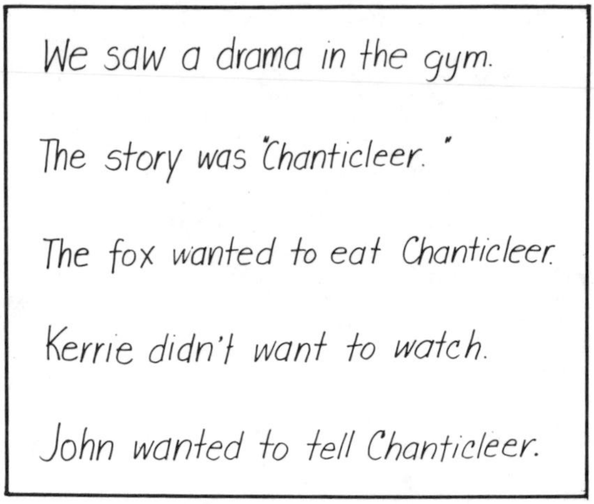

We saw a drama in the gym.

The story was "Chanticleer."

The fox wanted to eat Chanticleer.

Kerrie didn't want to watch.

John wanted to tell Chanticleer.

FIGURE 5.32 This chart not only contains sentences that tell what happened that day, but also sentences that tell how some of the children reacted to the event.

Because the teaching of basic sentence patterns is a central concern in the lower school, much of the chart work is designed to present and reinforce specific language constructions. If sentence patterns are the focus of a lesson, then there are certain ways in which the chart can be written to simplify the task of reading it. And, if the child's confidence in reading is to grow, it is also necessary to consider the possible obstacles in a chart's format which make the use of reading skills more difficult.

Sources of difficulty in reading a chart can range from simple, spatial presentation to general lack of structural cohesiveness. For example, some very early readers might be confused by sentences that do not end on the line on which they began. *(FIGURE 5.33)* In a year or two, however, the one-sentence-to-a-line format may even hinder reading. The child may not see a link between sentence one and two and read them as disconnected and unrelated events.

Young children find things generally more readable when they do not have to rely on

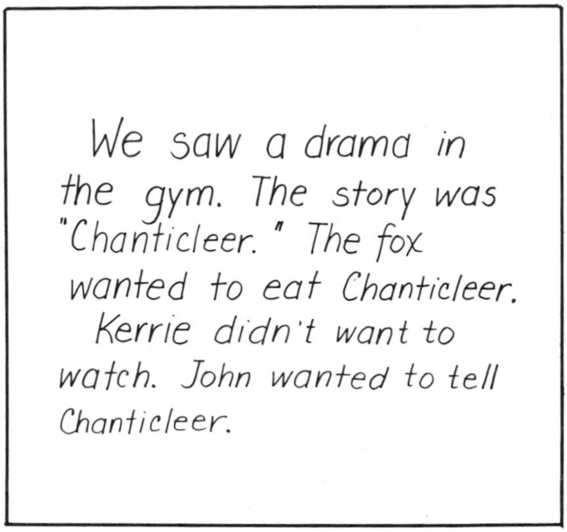

We saw a drama in
the gym. The story was
"Chanticleer." The fox
wanted to eat Chanticleer.
Kerrie didn't want to
watch. John wanted to tell
Chanticleer.

FIGURE 5.33 This chart is the same as that in Figure 5.32 except that the sentences do not all begin on the same line. This aids the teacher in developing reading fluency.

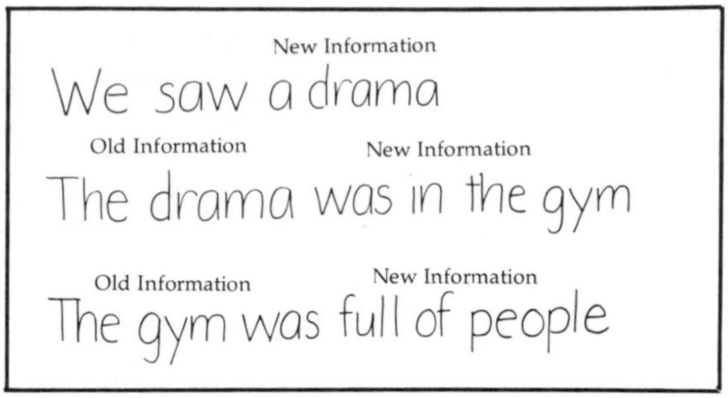

understanding every piece of textual data to glean the meaning of the story or chart. Experience-based charts facilitate understanding by depending upon the child's ability to remember classroom activity and reconstruct from what he knows of similar events.

Focus

Because linguistic structure is just becoming a true organizing tool for the beginning reader, it is important that the chart is structurally cohesive. Another important consideration in designing reading charts is the organizational tool of focus. In an experience chart, for example, many topics can become the object of focus. In the dramatic presentation of "Chanticleer and the Fox," a young child's focus can range from the crowd of people in the gym itself (a place he may normally see as quite different—light and rather empty) to the loudness of the actor's voices, to the actual dramatic action or one particular dramatic act.

Class discussion, illustrations of the events, and reenactments of the play can

New Information
We saw a drama
Old Information New Information
The drama was in the gym
Old Information New Information
The gym was full of people

FIGURE 5.34 Contrasting new and old information in reading materials is another aspect of developing reading comprehension.

handle much of the representation of experience, but a chart representing the entire experience would be very long and difficult to read.

A simple structural design following a topic-then-comment pattern is a useful teaching tool for directing the child's reading focus and for defining the central topics of the chart. Language structures are still apparent but the readability has been enhanced by constructing sentences which follow the old-then-new information pattern. The new information is introduced at the end of one sentence, but later becomes the old information at the beginning of the next sentence. *(FIGURE 5.34)*

Besides focusing the child's reading on central topics, this structural design is constructed for readability by helping students not to rely equally on each word of a sentence. By repeated use of simple sentences in a topic-then-comment pattern, a reader becomes fluent in predicting and anticipating content to be read.

Placing New Structures in the Chart

Presentation of structures for exposure and recognition is another consideration in designing more readable charts. Very often those language structures included in the reading chart for exposure and recognition purposes are not processed on any level. The reader should not have to depend on fully understanding the complex language structures to understand the chart story. Instead, he should rely on the context in which the new language is embedded or on his own knowledge of the story. For example, in the passage,

> Snow White ran into the woods *and* finally saw a cottage. The cottage was in the middle of a group of trees,

a student can use contextual clues, intonational clues or some anticipatory set to guess what the new conjoined *and* structure means. He does not have to read this conjoined sentence with the same weight he would read others.

The complexity of structures appearing for exposure or recognition purposes does not have to confound or stop the reading process. One of the roles of the chart's internal structural design is to ensure the active use of inductive and anticipatory skills.

Making Reading Materials

While aware of the interface between language and reading and the transfer of language skills to reading strategies, one cannot assume that this transfer is automatic. In the lower school years, reading strategies should become the object of direct instruction and can be developed using many of the same formats previously described. These formats should influence the organization of charts, workbooks, or in-class activities.

Reading skills can be defined here as highly specialized and fluent performances done by the reader. In the early years these performances depend on many variables: the child's purpose for reading, the task required of him by the teacher, and what the student perceives the reading task to be. For example, the young reader may sometimes see reading as a visual task and point out that the word *talk* looks like *walk* in the sentence "Roger Williams could not talk to the Indians," and *great* has an *eat* in it as in the book The Great Escape (Lippmann, 1973).

Reading may be interpreted as auditory contrast; the child may see that *try* sounds like *cry* and perceive this as a game to be played. Reading can also be mapping a whole word to a sign or gesture (quite often both performed with little attention to context). Or, if a question asked by the teacher is one that cannot be handled easily and demands interpretation, reading will be perceived as constructing relationships between known words in the sentence. Still for others, the task is clearly to get to the end of the sentence without stopping or being stopped by anything–sounds, words, or teachers.

The strangest phenomenon growing out of their efforts to read is that young children like what they are doing. They like to be called on to read; they often monitor themselves and refuse to let the class continue until they have it right. They are critical of others reading (jumping up to protest if a neighbor misses a word) and most importantly of all, they do not seem bothered by the fact that they really cannot tell you very much about what they have just read.

The children's own responses to the task at hand serve as an index for the teacher as to what reading skills they are ready to develop. Research shows that beginning readers are very limited in the amount of new words they can retain and recognize as well as how fluidly they can process old information using a letter-by-letter approach or an initial letter and guess strategy. Too often in classroom conversation, the child fingerspells the first letter of the word he wants to use or repeats vocally the initial sound. In the hurry of the classroom, where most content is commonly shared and understood (especially by the teacher), the isolated letter strategy seems efficient to the child.

The reading experiences at this level should develop and capitalize on the reader's skill of visually chunking spelling patterns together. In the phonic poem *(FIGURE 5.35)* the repetition of the *ight* and *ee* configurations and the sheer visual bombardment makes

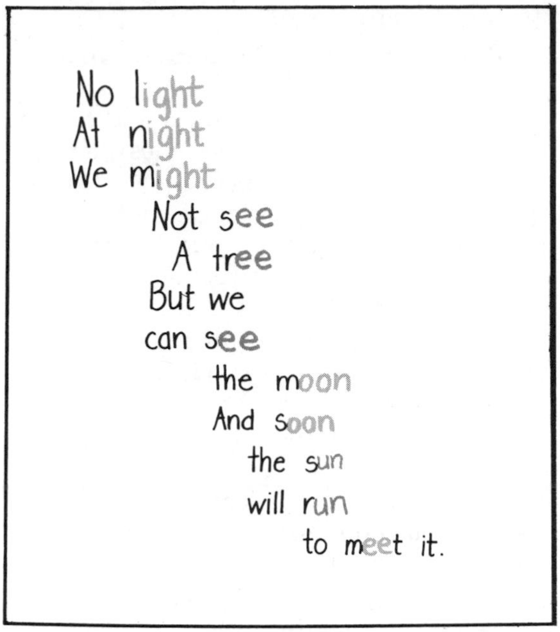

No light
At night
We might
Not see
A tree
But we
can see
the moon
And soon
the sun
will run
to meet it.

FIGURE 5.35 This phonic poem, presented in chart form, is used to develop both visual and auditory "chunking."

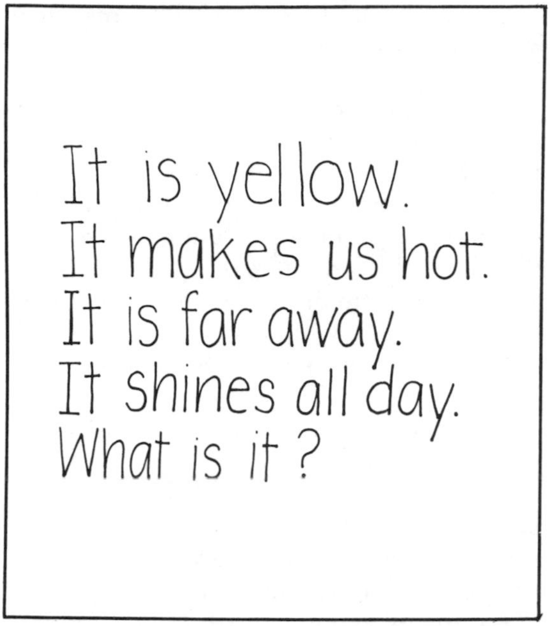

It is yellow.
It makes us hot.
It is far away.
It shines all day.
What is it?

FIGURE 5.36 Riddles are a good exercise to develop thinking and categorization by attribute.

chunking these patterns an automatic process after one or two lines. In this case, the child learns rather quickly that each letter must not necessarily be processed in isolation. If part of the reading process is skilled behavior, teachers should aim for greater automaticity and anticipation in the behaviors to be performed.

Research has shown that hearing-impaired readers use as much visual chunking as hearing readers. This strategy, as Fries (1966) suggests, should become a fundamental processing skill. Further workbook activities that supplement the reading of a story may make use of both visual groupings and semantic constraints. A cloze-phonic exercise is an example of such a workbook exercise.

The boy read the entire hook/book in one hour.

Riddles, a good reading activity, can help the child to develop categorizing skills and infer meaning beyond the text. As the context of attribute clues *(It is yellow)* and functional clues *(It shines)* grows, the child anticipates what the unknown referent might be while revising earlier guesses as informational constraints grow. Though this exercise may be difficult for the 7-year-old who is still in the preoperational stage (and cannot categorize in terms of more than one attribute), the child is still anxious to guess and learn to revise his guesses. *(FIGURE 5.36)*

USE OF BOOK FORMAT

In the lower school, use of book form for presentation of reading material is very important. The simple manipulation of the book itself is enjoyable to children. Turning pages back and forth from one picture to another is an active participation in reading which is lessened by the exclusive use of chart form.

Structurally, the book form lends itself well to building such reading strategies as prediction and anticipation. In a book like One Monday Morning by Uri Shulevitz (1967), for instance, all the *buts* appear before the reader turns the page, and they come at points when the reader is either waiting for or guessing what will come next. It is easy to see how this element of anticipation could be lost if this story were presented in chart form.

For those children who are being exposed to language structures in a chart form, such as conjoined sentences, reintroducing the story in book form after the action or story line is familiar can draw more attention to the conjunction *and* without demanding a full understanding of its syntactic function. The children's knowledge of the story, their anticipation and command of the events, facilitates their reading of the language.

Recently there are many books, formally classified as picture books, with a format generally consisting of pictures accompanied by one or two caption-like lines of text. Where the Wild Things Are (Sendak, 1963) and The Three Robbers (Ungerer, 1962) are examples of this format. Picture books such as these should remain around the room or in the reading area for children to reread over an extended period of time. At each reading the child brings something new to the book–a new purpose or a sense of success because he's read it before and knows what will happen. This sense of command over written material is a vital reinforcement. Too often once the actual reading text, chart, book or sentence strip is mastered, it disappears only to be replaced by new reading material. Although the teacher might refer back and draw analogies to previous information or stories read, the student does not necessarily draw the same analogies on his own. The teacher's references, then, become proof only of her good memory.

Small running libraries of stories and charts read in class should be accessible to the children for more than the brief span of a unit or topic. Such libraries help to emphasize one of the potentials of literature: its recyclability. Reading and rereading a story with a sense of accomplishment are reinforcing experiences for all young children.

THEORIES OF READING COMPREHENSION AND QUESTIONING

As the child moves into his third and fourth years of lower school, he becomes increasingly familiar with sentence types. This is when all the reading strategies which the student has been learning to use contribute more and more to his comprehension of the reading materials.

Because of the varieties of strategies that should be available to the child, the goals for comprehension should not be derived by looking at any one structural level alone. Restricting the scope of the reading process to knowledge of language constructions and their manipulation, for example, limits the possibilities of the student actively employing other processing skills while reading. Some of these skills the student naturally has been using; others, he has been taught to use. And whether work on developing reading skills has been integrated into charts and book forms, or into teacher-designed workbooks, demand for comprehension of story is steadily increasing. This demand is dictated by both the complexity of text, the reader's motivation and other reading tasks established by the teacher.

Comprehension Defined

Some investigators have said that understanding what you read is in some way isomorphic to thinking. To paraphrase Gibson and Levin (1975, p. 400), in order to comprehend the meaning of a word, a sentence, or a story, one must be able to follow the thinking of the writer and, at the same time, interpolate and extrapolate in order to get the full meaning intended. One must, then, be able to infer, to problem-solve, to deduct, etc.

The notion that reading is thinking is clearly reflected in models of comprehension. These models isolate specific levels at which meaning can be acquired, while delineating specific component skills necessary to this comprehension. Modeling their descriptions

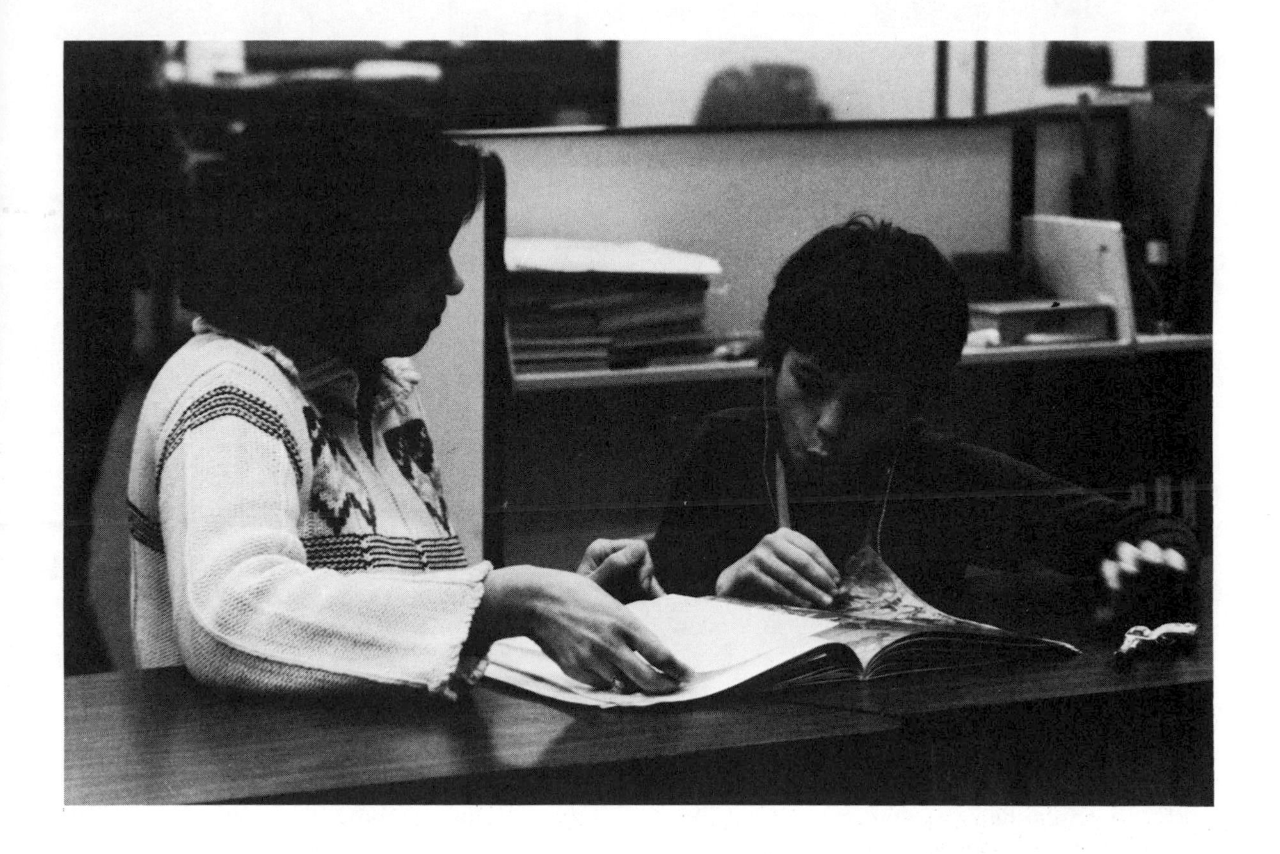

on those of Guilford's (1960) "structure of the intellect," researchers have devised lengthy taxonomies of reading comprehension covering a broad range of skills. After decades of debate over which skills from one theorist's list were distinct from skills of another's list (Herber, 1970; Bond & Wagner, 1966; Gans, 1963), studies by F. B. Davis (1968) have statistically isolated critical comprehension skills. *(FIGURE 5.38)*

In most cases, component skill lists such as this are the organizational core around which classroom reading and its assessment revolve. One simply has to look at the most recent teacher's guides in basal reading systems to discover that judging how well a child understands what he is reading is determined by how many literal, inferential and evaluative skills he has. Many educators feel that these levels of comprehension are actual

READING COMPREHENSION SUBSKILLS

1. Recalling word meanings from context
2. Inferring about word meaning
3. Answering explicit questions from text
4. Weaving together ideas in context
5. Drawing inferences from text
6. Recognizing writer's purpose
7. Identifying a writer's technique
8. Following structure of a passage

Source: Adapted from F.B. Davis, "Research in Reading," *Reading Research Quarterly,* Summer, 1968, *3*, p. 499-545.

FIGURE 5.38 Reading comprehension subskills

sequences in the process of reading comprehension and are therefore useful in measuring it. It seems clear, however, from the most recent perceptual, linguistic and psycholinguistic research that these levels of comprehension simply are not accurate indices of the processes which underlie the comprehension of meaning and cannot be used as models for assessing reading comprehension.

Bormuth et al. (1970) examined children's abilities to answer questions which focus on syntactic units. By basing their investigation on transformational questions limited to the syntactic level, they intended to use the theory of transformational-generative grammar to develop a systematic theory of comprehension. However their fourth grade subjects could not successfully answer seemingly simple *wh*-questions about isolated sentences and the researchers were left with explaining the results. Other research has shown that answering questions involves more than the manipulation of syntactic constituents. If the question/answer format is used in reading work, the teacher must often go beyond the sentence level to extended text.

Evaluation of Comprehension: Questioning

Questioning a child about a story is different from teaching the question forms. When one's goal is comprehension, one must question whether or not the reader understood the meaningful or most central structures of the story; the characters' motives, the location of the crucial climactic act, the resolution, or what happened at the end. The focus and task should be one of evaluating comprehension of text and diagnosing where reading strengths and weaknesses lie.

As reading research has indicated (Gibson & Levin, 1975), much less is known about how one processes and comprehends extended text. It is difficult to define the units of information which constitute a passage of discourse and models of comprehension offered by reading theorists have yet to accommodate reading of text.

J. Carroll and R. Freedle (1972) respond to the problem of having to devise a specific model of comprehension by proposing that perhaps it is the function of the question which demands closer attention. The distinction between literal processing and higher level processing becomes clearer in the teacher's use of the question/answer format. Carefully designed literal questions set the task to be performed and delineate the elements within the text from which they are derived. The question controls and limits the textual information which can be used in its response.

Questions should not exclusively assess literal recall skills, however. In a study by Guszak (1967), which analyzed the oral questioning strategies of 12 elementary school teachers, it was found that over 60 percent of teachers' questions focused on these literal recall skills. Little effort was made in requiring children to draw inferences from and make judgments about the text or to justify their responses. This type of classroom questioning reflects a confusion on the teacher's part or on the program's part; a reading skill (the ability to identify the relevant semantic elements of the text) is being mistaken as a reading ability (thinking about these elements in a certain way) (Parker, 1969).

In many ways teachers are not even assessing reading skills or comprehension. Rather, they are simply measuring the child's memory or his ability to manipulate the surface structures of a question by matching its constituents to those in the text. Children often use strategies which defeat the purpose of testing comprehension, especially the hearing-impaired child who tends to overuse these strategies. In a passage such as,

> The boy saw it all happen. The room shook. Vases shattered. A mist clouded the windows.

answering the question "What did the boy see?" with "It all happen" is a poor strategy.

Looking at a teacher's guide to a basal reading series, one finds that a majority of the questions requires the child to search for a sentence in the passage with the same elements as the question and then substitute the *wh* pro-form (*who, what, where*) for the appropriate constituents. This requires an automatic response to grammatical transformation; attention need not be paid to the meaning of the question or the text.

Not only is the level of questioning superficial, but the sequencing of questions does not recognize the possibilities within the questioning process for guiding and extending inferential treatment of the text. Nor does it recognize that narrative structures cannot be parsed and questioned in a rigid, sequential manner. Reading story charts requires responding to information and detail. Because this information exists within a context governed by form, questions asked must take into account the interpretive aspects, which are part of responding to literature. It is the method of questioning which can refine this important response.

EXPOSURE TO LITERARY FORM IN LOWER SCHOOL

A sense of accomplishment is crucial for the early reader. Without this sense, however different it is from an adult's, future reading by the student may be undermined.

One of the tools that assures success is the reader's reliance on forms of literary text (fairy tales, rhymes, prose fiction) and the structural elements inherent within these forms (character, action, and plot). Exposing the child to these reading forms and structures can provide the reader with much needed success and commitment to reading, and maintaining exposure to literary forms within the school curriculum helps to amplify the child's recognition of structures within stories. These forms and structures can then be compared by the reader so that eventually he develops a sense of story which generates or goes beyond those stories which he has read or has had read to him.

Both reading and writing demand a sense of structure.

"Even a little child must come to learn what stories are before he likes listening to them. He has, in fact, to develop a rudimentary poetics [structure] of fiction before he learns to respond just as he develops a grammatical sense in order to speak" (Scholes, 1974, p. 130).

The lower school child may not have all the linguistic structures and reading strategies needed to independently read many of the literary forms, particularly short stories which he might naturally select. The reading experiences must include exposure to forms, such as stories and poems, read or told to the student by someone who does have the reading ability.

"One essential aspect of literary training, and one that it is possible to acquire or begin acquiring in lower school, is the art of listening to stories and poetry. This sounds like a passive ability, but it is not passive at all. It is what the army would call a basic training for the imagination" (Frye [in Sloan, 1975, p. 75]).

Although one would hope that story telling, nursery rhymes, and games would be part of the young child's home situation, teachers cannot assume that the lower school learner comes with the simplest concepts of speaker-receiver relationships. Thus, story telling, retelling, listening, watching and responding are behaviors that very often must be worked at during the school years.

Initially the young reader or listener is captivated by action-oriented structures of stories and poems. Plot takes a back seat to the events occurring within the frame. The type of characters found in these stories are cardboard caricatures of real people. Thus, there is the mean farmer's wife in the rhyme "Three Blind Mice," or the hen in the story "The Little Red Hen." Characters, both animals and people, seem to be suspended in an arbitrary frame of events that succeed in captivating the early reader.

These stereotyped caricatures should quickly make room for one of the cornerstones of future work in reading: the archetypal character. The archetype, the hero or good guy, and the antihero or bad guy are the first types of characters actually affected by the action and plot of a story. The plot structures themselves, at this time, are also archetypal and deal with universal themes: either the journey (Where the Wild Things Are), the completion of some task (The Little Engine That Could), or the triumphant return (Jack the Giant Killer).

In the lower school years, the young reader will prefer action plots with little character motivation. Archetypal characters are not considered cardboard at all by the young reader and, although exposed to stories with more character intervention, the readers' own choices will be of texts with simple plots and structural redundancy. For example, simple forms of poetry with recursive choral frames (such as "Old MacDonald Had A Farm") contribute to the early reader's apprehension of structural elements in his reading strategies.

The elements in a story on which a child may capitalize are always evolving. Therefore, it is important that in class discussion and questioning the teacher considers the story the young reader has read, not the story the teacher has read, even though the titles may be the same.

In structurally simple stories, the repetitive action still monopolizes the reader's attention and questions dealing with possible character motivation elicit confusion or indifference. Repeated questioning by the teacher and her discounting of the student's inappropriate answers can frustrate both teacher and student. Although the student likes and understands the story, he is simply unable to come up with the answer the teacher wants.

Reading in the early years should not be confined to simple action-plot stories, but the timing of the move to more complex story forms and structures is one that must be well conceived and meaningfully prepared for by the teacher. When it is time for students to move from simple action to holding in tension both the action and the action altered by the intervention of some archetypal character, careful classroom discussion is sometimes the teacher's best friend. In these stories, action does not proceed as randomly and character motivation is more an inherent part of the story structure (e.g., "Icarus and Daedalus", or "King Midas"). James Moffett recognizes the potential for classroom discussion as a pattern for learning in A Student-Centered Language Arts Curriculum K-6 (1973).

Discussion is a process of amending, appending, diverging, converging, elaborating, summarizing, and many other things. Most of all, it is an external social process that each member gradually internalizes as a personal thought process: he begins to think in the ways his group talks. Not only does he take unto himself the vocabulary, usage, and syntax of others and synthesize new creations out of their various styles, points of view, and attitudes, he also structures his thinking into mental operations resembling the operations of the group interactions. If the group amends, challenges, elaborates, and qualifies together, each member begins to do so alone in his inner speech" (p. 46).

From this point on, story structure becomes one of more personalized characterization and more cohesive plot construction. Characters intervene to meaningfully change the chain of events and their motivations and consequences become much more apparent. Rudimentary parallel plot construction and plot completions can now build on the child's attention to story structure. These activities help the child to see how conflicts are resolved by some climactic act or character intervention. Relying on structures allows the reader to predict or anticipate events in a story.

There are indications that hearing-impaired children are handling more of the elements of literature than teachers realize. A group of 7-year-olds reading "The Christmas Carol" proved this point. Not only did they respond to the high-interest level of the plot and the action of the story, but recalling the story months later they identified with their favorite characters. Scrooge, hated by them all, became the archetypal antihero and in discussing him the children expressed opinions about selfishness and greed. In fact, the children learned the term *selfishness* through this story. In classroom discussion they used the word *scrooge* in novel and sometimes unexpected ways. Such use is vital in that

> *"it is able to turn to use those mysterious, grotesque, creepy, crepuscular, iridescent experiences which the child generally feels he had better leave outside the school door, but which obsess him and rob his attention"* (Lopate, 1976, p. 331).

SUGGESTED READINGS

READING AND LITERATURE

Arbuthnot, M.H. *The Arbuthnot anthology of children's literature.* Glenview: Scott, Foresman & Co., 1971.

Arbuthnot, M.H. & Sutherland, Z. *Children and books.* Glenview: Scott, Foresman & Co., 1972.

Chomsky, C. Write now, read later. In C. Cazden (Ed.), *Language in early childhood education.* Washington, D.C.: National Association for the Education of Young Children, 1972.

Everetts, E. (Ed.). *Explorations in children's writing.* Chaplain, IL: National Council of Teachers of English, 1970.

Huck, C., & Kuhn, D. *Children's literature in the elementary school.* New York: Holt, Rinehart & Winston, 1966.

Koch, K. *Wishes, Lies and Dreams.* New York: Chelsea House, 1970.

Koch, K. *Rose, where did you get that red?* New York: Vintage Books, 1973.

Kohl, H. *Reading, how to.* New York: Bantam Books, 1973.

ACKNOWLEDGMENTS

FIGURES

Page 75 *Figure 5.28* Class by Susan Kondas, Rhode Island School for the Deaf. Photograph courtesy of Ira Garber.

Page 81 *Figure 5.30* From unit prepared by Mary Weiner and Peter Geisser, Rhode Island School for the Deaf. Photograph courtesy of Ira Garber.

Page 81 *Figure 5.31* From unit prepared by Ann-Marie Clarkson, Rhode Island School for the Deaf.

Page 85 *Figure 5.35* Chart prepared by Deborah Topol, Rhode Island School for the Deaf.

Page 85 *Figure 5.36* From unit prepared by Leslie Williams, Rhode Island School for the Deaf.

Chapter 6

Introduction to Complexity

The period of curriculum work utilizing primarily simple sentence structures, although painfully slow, corresponds closely to the observable cognitive development of the child. However, with the development of complex language, issues of cognition also become complex and difficult to identify.

The years from eight to eleven are crucial ones for language development in the hearing-impaired child. It is during this period that the acquisition of complex sentence structures is both possible and necessary since the growth of complex syntax is inextricably related to the growing complexity of the cognitive tasks confronted both in school and elsewhere. Concurrently, as demands for more involved social communication arise, more complex reading performance and written expression are necessary. If syntactic ability, both receptive and expressive, limits a student's response to these types of demands, then clearly the expansion of syntactic competence during this period must be one goal of a language development curriculum.

However, there is at this stage the possibility of two factors occurring in the teaching process which need to be avoided. The first factor is the failure to see that a child's cognitive development involves the development of a coherent and integrated system–one which effectively organizes the world around him. Piaget refers to the child as being in the subperiod of concrete operations during which there is a rapid growth in the child's organization of his context. If the child's organizing process is to be effective, sufficient data and experiences are required. Not all children at this stage will be organizing in precisely the same way or to the same degree of complexity. The teacher needs to be diagnostic about the child by observing the kinds of strategies he is using to organize information. Most importantly, the methods used by teachers in the classroom should be sensitive to the students' organizational processes.

Of possible help at this point is an analysis of some children's written productions about a picture of a birthday party held in a garage because of rain.

The first sample *(FIGURE 6.39)* is a simple description of various activities in the picture. The syntax is also simple in its structure. The language is really an extension of the naming (or referencing) process using basic simple sentences. Furthermore, the sentences are random observations with little sequence.

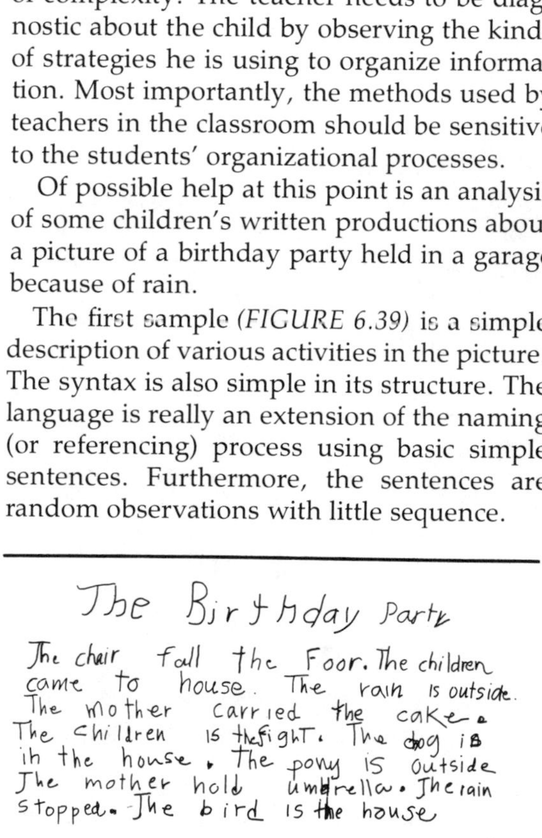

The Birthday Party

The chair fall the Foor. The children came to house. The rain is outside. The mother carried the cake. The children is the fight. The dog is in the house. The pony is outside. The mother hold umbrella. The rain stopped. The bird is the house

Figure 6.39

The second example (FIGURE 6.40) indicates a significant shift in the organizational (operational) abilities of the child. The sentences are not random; there is a sense of awareness of the event as a whole and there is also a sensitivity to the causal and relational factors within the event.

The BirtHDaY PaRTY

We had a birthday party in the garage, because it's rainy today. They think, "they should not ride a pony outside. The pony was sad. The children began to fool and fight "because it's rainy." The boy punched boy's nose. Two women came out of the door. There are five candles on the cake. The girl pat the kitten. The boy looked down at the kitten. The children got fun!

Figure 6.40

The issue here is not only the difference in language but a difference in the cognitive processes observable in the writing. To be able to talk and write about causal relationships requires not only the cognitive skill itself, but the language structures as well.

The second factor that presents itself as a possible problem is the shift in teaching style that often occurs at this level. The teacher, intuitively aware that students are more sophisticated cognitively than linguistically, attempts to teach complex linguistic structures in a formal, artificial or prescriptive manner. It is important, therefore, for the teacher to recognize that the process of language development at this stage of complexity is no different than that of early language acquisition. Structures are to be acquired, not taught, and before any discussion or analysis of such structures is held there should be a period of meaningful exposure to them. If the teacher is aware of the language needs of the student and sensitive to what the next stage of development might be, then almost any subject matter can become the vehicle for introducing new complex structures.

Two major considerations are involved in determining how to bring complex thinking and language into the classroom. Firstly, the cognitive level of the students must be taken into account, particularly in choosing appropriate materials. Secondly, there are aspects of the form and function of particular syntactic and semantic structures to be considered. Before returning to more practical examples it will be useful to discuss these cognitive and linguistic considerations.

Complexity and Cognitive Growth

The 8- to 10-year-old child is moving from event sequencing to a more complex conception of space, time and causality. Accordingly, the language work should reflect that growth and change. Questions of causality involving more than one event are introduced, with the ordering of events playing a greater role. Following the mastery of the relationship of events in a given context, the child may begin focusing on the attributes of things within the events, and during this period may even lose track of the events themselves.

A crucial aspect of cognitive development is the shift from concreteness to operationality as reflected in conservation (see Chapter 2). The development of conservation will enable the child to handle both event and attribute in relation to each other, to the extent of understanding that often intrinsic, causal relationships exist between the attributes of people (or characters in stories) and events that occur (or plot). This cognitive growth opens up the possibility for meaningful use of literature in the classroom. In fact, a decreasing emphasis on event orientation and an increasing ability to reference attributes in relation to events are critical to the development of reading skills and abilities.

Syntactic and Semantic Complexity

The hearing-impaired child enters this period with a sense for the simple sentence grammar of English and the beginnings of syntactic complexity. In the previous developmental stage, the student has already been exposed to and hopefully has acquired several keys to the expansion of syntactic complexity. Simple verb conjunction (Kelly jumped *and* played.) should have been mastered as well as infinitive noun phrase complements appearing in the verb phrase, (John likes *to read books*). The student who comes out of the simple sentence stage with a mastery of basic simple sentence patterns, comprehension of infinitive noun phrase complements, and the roots of conjunction is ready for a program involving syntactic complexity.

One factor that necessitates the move to complexity is the increased demand for functional language. Much more is expected communicatively and linguistically from the 9-year-old child than from the preschooler. The ability to explain or reference one's own actions, the actions of friends or to relate the day's events to a parent requires surprisingly complex syntactic and semantic abilities.

For instance, after her daughter's two-day camping trip, the mother of one 11-year-old reported that all her daughter told her about the trip was "far, far, far." Certainly there was much more information to relate but to do so would have required some complex language structures involving time, distance and reference, particularly in describing events and people. When one party in a conversation has not experienced the same events as the other, as in the case of the mother trying to learn about her daughter's camping experience, the ability to reference and relate events and relationships is essential. Without this ability, communication breaks down. Syntactically, clause embeddings, common to indirect discourse as well as to other complex syntactic and semantic processes, are necessary in this situation.

Three syntactic processes involved in the generation of complex sentences are discussed in this chapter:

conjunction

subordination (adverbial clauses)
(relative clauses)

simple sentence transformation

Conjunction

During the earlier school years the student will have developed a notion of simple conjunction processes. This will, in general, have begun in the verb phrase (Sheila laughed *and* giggled), moved to all noun phrase positions (Bill *and* Sue picked flowers), and perhaps moved on to conjunction of simple sentences, usually with *and* (Kelly jumped *and* Cari skipped). In fact, it is a common observation that many young children string together inappropriately long sequences of simple sentences using one all-purpose connector. Often this process begins with the use of a sentence-initial connector that appears almost at random in the child's connected language productions.

Involved in this process is the developing sense of ordering and sequencing of events reflected in various forms of conjunction such as:

	SENTENCE 1.		SENTENCE 2.
a.	King Midas touched his plate.		It turned to gold.
b.	King Midas touched his plate.	[And then / And / Then / So]	it turned to gold.
c.	King Midas touched his plate	[and then / and / then / so]	it turned to gold.

The sense for conjoining reflected in (b) is helped by the tone of voice and stress utilized in the story-telling process. An atmosphere of anticipation is created by the effective use of "and then . . . "

If hearing-impaired children are to adequately master conjoining, they too need to share in the anticipation of story telling. The power of the stressed conjunction is a valuable speech activity and can be highlighted by

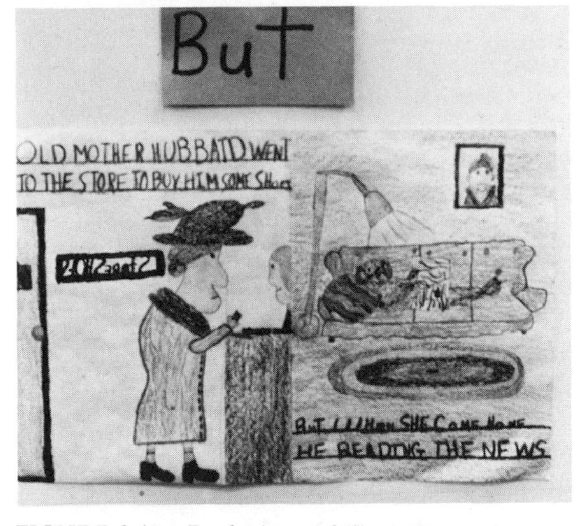

FIGURE 6.41 Producing and illustrating sentences conjoined by but *aids students in mastering this form of conjunction.*

reading such stories as "The Old Woman and the Pig" or "The Little Red Hen." Practice should help the child utilize (c) in which there is anticipation of events in sequence.

Where the connector is *because* or *so*, the strung-together sentences are representations of events related by cause and effect, time, sequence or other possible organizing principles. Two examples from a language lesson based on a camping experience illustrate this difference:

a. **Simple sentence conjunction; event orientation:**
Some boys cut wood *and* some boys cleaned the canoes.

b. **Simple sentence conjunction; relational:**
We built a fire *and then* we roasted marshmallows.

A number of experiments (Sinclair-de-Zwart, 1969) point out the differences in the language of conserving and nonconserving children. For example, nonconservers tend to use simple, one-dimensional conjunctions (This dog is big and this dog is small), while children with a functioning sense of conservation tend to use more relationally complex conjunctions (This dog is big but not as big as this one).

It is important to recognize the difference between simple conjunction and relational conjunction. Simple conjunction connects two events or sentences but does not really specify a relationship between them as in,

We saw lions *and* we saw tigers.

Relational conjunction, on the other hand, specifies a certain semantic relationship between the conjoined sentences and may require one sentence to be subordinated to the other. The following are examples of some of the different types of relational conjunction:

The clowns were funny *but* the tigers were scary.
The Queen was beautiful *but* wicked.
It rained *so* we came home.

Subordination: Adverbial Clauses

Certain adverbial clause structures describe a variety of event-ordering relationships rather than a strict sequencing of conjunctional structures, such as,

a. [When / Before / After] you finish your math, (SENTENCE 1 (EVENT 1),) you may go to lunch. (SENTENCE 2 (EVENT 2).)

b. You may go to lunch (SENTENCE 1) [when / before / after] you finish your math. (SENTENCE 2)

Teachers often see these adverbials as reflections of time concepts rather than as relationships that can speak of either past, present or future events.

a. Before you go to lunch, you will finish your math. (future)
b. Before you went to lunch, you finished your math. (past)

It may be more manageable for the teacher to use enactive and iconic experiences to introduce the *before* and *after* structures such as in number ordering;

Before 4 is 3.
After 5 is 6.

This process can also be used with plot diagrams that outline the events of a story. Adverbials, however, are more than event-ordering structures in that they also reflect concepts of causality.

SENTENCE 1		SENTENCE 2.
(EVENT 1)	so	(EVENT 2)
Gretel cried	because	she was lost.

Some linguists identify this type of *because* or *so* structure as conjoined because it seems more like a coordinated sentence than a subordinate clause/main clause. As conjoining and adverbial clause work can overlap in the acquisition process, this argument should not be a problem for the teacher who chooses to identify it in the way best suited to a particular group of children.

As children become comfortable with processing a number of events and the sequential relationships between them, they should be developing an increasing awareness of the causal relationship between the events in response to the *why* question form.

Relative Clauses

The difficulty that hearing-impaired children have with the relative clause structure is well documented by Quigley et al. (1976) and it is a commonly observed phenomenon that students tend to interpret *wh*–relativizers and other *wh*–subordinators as question words. The child who is routinely processing *wh*–words as indicators that a question is being asked needs to formulate a wider generalization or linguistic rule. *Wh*–words are major signals of embedded sentences which describe and/or relate the major semantic force of the matrix sentence to another sentence, or even to another unmentioned attribute or place such as,

"Boston is the city *where I was born*."

Therefore, the child's linguistic competence must expand to syntactically and semantically process these *wh*–words and the clauses that follow them as attribute statements, not as direct questions. The move from work on *wh*–words as question markers to *wh*–words as relative or other subordinate clause markers is a point where most traditional language programs falter. Thus, in addition to complexity in reference and increasing sophistication in conjunction, description as in relative and other *wh*–clauses is a major area of complex syntactic development.

The relative clause structure is one that a teacher can build into almost any language activity. One teacher, when classifying vertebrates and invertebrates, utilized the relative clause as part of the classifying process:

"Invertebrates are animals *that have no backbone*."

Another teacher, as part of a unit on values development, chose to do a series of fables with the intent of discussing the moral of each fable. Her story of "The Boy Who Cried Wolf" began with,

Peter was a boy *who lived in a castle*.

The relative clause was used from time to time throughout each fable thereby exposing the students to a common complex structure and at the same time giving the teacher the added descriptive power of the relative clause with which to keep the fables interesting.

Another teacher was doing a social studies project on early American colonial life. The subtopic began with a presentation by the teacher of the general classification of craftsmen, followed by a more intensive study of several colonial crafts. These activities provided an ideal vehicle for the presentation of relative clauses.

The particular project on crafts lasted four weeks and out of the classroom experiences came such sentences as,

A blacksmith was a craftsman *who worked with iron*.

Children *who were old enough* helped in the shop.

People respected craftsmen *who were skillful*.

By exposing her students to these structures in the context of a fully developed unit, and through comprehension work in the same context, the teacher is able to make these structures accessible and meaningful for them. The same kind of internalizing activity that was seen at the simple sentence level is therefore involved at this more complex level. In addition, the stage can be set for reading comprehension and written and verbal production of these structures.

Simple Sentence Transformation: Passive Voice

The passive voice structure, which changes a sentence such as "Lucy hit Charlie Brown" to "Charlie Brown was hit by Lucy," is very difficult to introduce meaningfully in a classroom setting. Firstly, it is not clear when and why it is mastered by hearing children. Menyuk (1969) makes reference to the passive-like structure (Sally got hit), which seems to appear at an early age. Quigley and Power (1973) show the difficulty that hearing-impaired children have with this sentence type. Specifically, hearing-impaired children tend to utilize semantic information and interpret it in terms of actor-action-object thereby misunderstanding the meaning of the passive voice. Secondly, the tendency in the classroom is to teach the passive voice mechanically, transforming active into passive sentences by supplying an object and subject, adding a helping auxiliary, changing the verb tense and adding a preposition.

Consideration of several factors will be helpful in determining when and how the passive might be introduced formally.

(1) Is it immediately useful? That is, is there some pragmatic reason why it should be introduced? Does it occur in a basal reader? Does the occurrence of awkward structures indicate the student's attempt to use the passive construction?

A teacher asked one 10-year-old child a question about the King Midas story which had been recently read in class. The student replied, "When the princess gave the food she said 'Thank you.' " This production might have been either the result of not understanding social etiquette or a general language inefficiency. The teacher asked the student to dramatize the sentence. It then became obvious that the student's intention was to use the passive, but as the syntactic structure was not known, the past tense word *gave* was used instead of *was given*. This seemed an appropriate time to introduce the new form.

(2) Are there some activities in the classroom which lend themselves well to introducing the passive?

One teacher happened to be discussing great inventors.

Alexander Graham Bell invented the telephone.
The telephone was invented by Alexander Graham Bell.
The Wright Brothers invented the airplane.
The airplane was invented by the Wright Brothers.

If it is necessary to formally describe the changes that occur in the transformational process, immediate advantage should be taken of the opportunity to read or use the forms in a meaningful context.

Several cautionary factors need to be kept in mind while doing the passive.

a. Nonreversible passives where the object is not likely to act on the subject (the telephone cannot invent Alexander Graham Bell) are easier to work with than reversible passives where semantically either subject or object can be an actor (Charlie Brown was hit by Lucy).

b. Pronouns and verb forms can be a problem in active to passive transformations, as seen in sentence e.

1. She hit Charlie Brown
2. Charlie Brown was hit by her.
3. Bill gave him an artichoke.
4. An artichoke was given him by Bill.
5. Him was given an artichoke by Bill.

c. It is common for agent deletion to occur in a passive sentence.

1. Fred threw the ball hard.
2. The ball was thrown hard by Fred.
3. The ball was thrown hard.

A CASE STUDY: TROLLS

The ideas and suggestions of the preceding sections can be illustrated by describing a unit taught to a group of students just beginning to move from the event level to attribute orientation. All of these children understood and produced simple sentences, although there was a variation in both their oral and written language.

Their language work up to this point included analysis of simple sentence patterns, comprehension of all types of question forms, simple adverbs and adjectives, negatives, imperatives and prepositional phrases which were for the most part event oriented. They had covered most of the transformations that operate on simple sentences and had also been exposed to more complex language, both in chart stories and in the reading program. At this stage they are ready for specific exposure to the complex syntactic and semantic structures needed to move on to another level of cognitive, linguistic and educational functioning.

At their present level these students are event oriented and respond primarily to the action in a story. Their major mode of response is to recreate the action of the story by acting it out. It is difficult for them to discuss reasons for or consequences of events in a story, or to express more than a "didn't like" or "liked it" opinion about the story or any of its characters.

It is important to recognize that an evaluative judgment is the earliest type of reading response and indicates that the young reader lacks the language and reading tools necessary to allow his responses to be more comparative. Also it should be kept in mind that young children generally like what they know best and are tentative about less familiar material even though fascinated by it. Young children are aware of the most salient and obvious attributes of characters but are unable to draw conclusions about characters based on these attributes. In other words, they are not using implicit information in responding to written text.

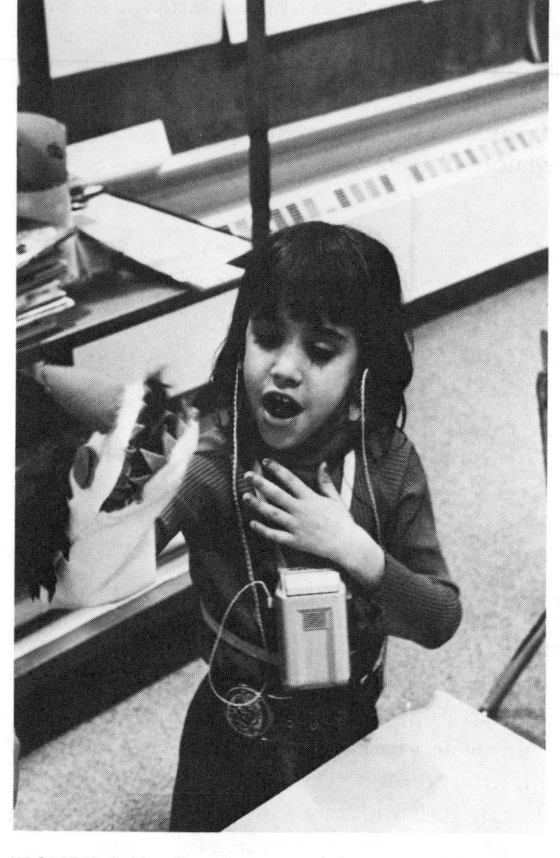

FIGURE 6.42 Reenactment of the story, "The Three Billy Goats Gruff"

For these reasons one teacher chose to use fairy tales, particularly troll stories, as the literary component and basis for her language work. Troll stories have the advantage of combining action, additive sequences of events and a few salient character attributes in each story. But the trolls have many shared characteristics no matter what the story.

One book that proved very useful, particularly for working on orientation to attribute, was Trolls by M. D'Aulaire (1975). This book contains not only event-oriented stories but descriptions characterizing many types of trolls. All of the examples that follow are from these stories.

One of the first activities of the unit was reading the troll story, "The Three Billy Goats Gruff," a story with repetitive action and very little descriptive language or characterization. The students were required to recreate the story by dramatization, an activity to which most children are very receptive. *(FIGURE 6.42)* Later, each student was asked to retell the story and the individual versions were written out, duplicated and given to the other students. The students told the story in basically simple sentences, but through some expansion and extension of their responses the rewritten story contained some conjoined sentences and adverbial clauses.

In addition to choosing stories with appropriate content for the cognitive level of the students, the teacher should set language goals which will support and enhance the growth of organizational and reading skills. Three areas of language development, previously discussed in terms of their relationship to cognition, were chosen as focal points of the language component of this unit. The language goals chosen were conjunction, adverbial clauses, and relative clauses.

(1) **Conjunction**

> The goats were on the bridge *and* the trolls were under the bridge.

This is the simplest type of conjoining; the sequencing of relationships requires no changes in the sentences but simply represents the joining of two events that occurred simultaneously. The next step might be to present sentences where there is referencing through pronominalization.

> The goats were on the bridge and the trolls were under *it*.

A third step might be deletion from the second sentence.

> The maidens wept and sobbed and (*they*) never expected to see the light of day again.

This construction can be presented to a class with a wide range of language abilities, allowing for different goals to be set for different students while keeping the same general class objectives. Eventually these students will need more complex relational conjunction (e.g., *but, because*) to expand the kinds of relationships they can comprehend and represent linguistically.

(2) **Adverbial Clauses**

The need for adverbial clauses to express causal and temporal relationships, which the children do in fact comprehend, is illustrated by contrasting a sentence taken from the troll story with a student's sentence.

> *Sentence from the story:* After the goat crushed the troll, he ate the grass.
>
> *Sentences from the child:* The goat crushed the troll. The goat ate the grass.

The student may have comprehended the relationship expressed in the original sentence but may lack the expressive skills needed to communicate this understanding. In this case, the teacher supplied the adverbial clause structure in the written version and used the student's simple sentence productions as a basis for helping him move toward a more complex system of expression.

(3) **Relative Clauses**

As discussed earlier, one of the syntactic structures necessary for the move to attribute orientation is the relative clause. Here are some examples of some relative clauses that appear in the troll stories.

> The mountains belonged to the trolls *who were as old and moss-grown as the mountains themselves.*
>
> Biggest and strongest of the trolls were those *who lived in the mountains.*
>
> *The trolls who had ribbons pinned to their knots* were the highest of the high.

One of the unit's activities was to compile a long list of troll attributes as they appeared in the stories. The list was displayed in class and was headed by the question, "What do you know about trolls?" Among the student responses to the first two stories were:

The troll mother was jealous.
The human mother was scared.
The troll was ugly.
The troll felt sorry.
The mother trolls traded babies.
The troll baby cried.
The troll has bugs in his hair.

Note that many of the responses are not attributes at all but rather events from the stories. In fact, out of the first twelve student responses collected, only four were actually attributes of trolls. From these responses, however, and by using sentences from the students' retold stories, the teacher began illustrating the embedding of one sentence in another by means of a relative clause. Using the children's productions shown above, the teacher and class were able to derive the following sentences:

The troll mother *who was jealous* traded babies.
The human mother *who spanked the baby troll* was scared.

This procedure allowed the teacher not only to begin work on relative clauses, but also to relate both the event and attribute sentences that the children themselves had produced.

Since these children produce and comprehend simple sentences, it is possible and effective to use these sentences to introduce relative clause structures. It must be clearly illustrated that a relative clause structure contains two simple sentences with an identical noun phrase, and that the relative pronoun refers to the preceding noun phrase. Language analysis can be used very effectively here to kernelize sentences containing relative clauses and to illustrate the embedding process. Other language teaching techniques, such as oral modeling, do not reveal the underlying structure of the sentence and they sometimes can be very unnatural, especially with complex sentence structures. One goal of the work on relative clauses is to help the students move away from interpreting all *wh-* words as question markers and move toward the understanding of *wh-* words as functioning to introduce modifying clauses. Other linguistic processes, such as pronominalization, are related to the three structures previously described and can be effectively presented along with those particular structures.

A Structural Approach to Reading and Literature

The levels of competence in reading literature are determined by many factors: individual literary preferences, linguistic development, experience with various forms of literature and general cognitive and psychological readiness. As the previous section has stressed, if students are to progress beyond a third grade reading level, the ability to understand more complex language structures is critical. One may read texts which use language structures such as relative clauses, coordinate clauses and adverbials, yet the level of reading will also be governed by cognitive demands made by isolated linguistic structures and by the structures inherent in the text or story as a whole. Structures in this context can range from recurring plot forms and character types, to stylistic devices that organize the text, to thematic structures.

The levels of reader competence, then, will in part be influenced by the structures that the student can bring to the work as well as by the generativity of the student's system for organizing elements of the texts read. For example, a generative reading ability will enable one to read and respond to fundamental patterns within specific stories as well as to generalize these principles to other previously read or soon-to-be-read materials of similar form and function.

Teachers of English in the middle school grades should focus on both an affect-centered approach and on an analytical approach. The more structures or systems of organization a child can use while reading literature, the more he will enjoy his reading experiences. Because reading is not solely dependent on language skills, and because the structures which organize text become more complex in more sophisticated literary forms, the teacher's role in selecting, rewriting or questioning reading materials becomes critical. Only through selecting or devising cohesively designed texts can complex literary structures become functional in developing reading skills.

Given the many levels of competence or understanding on which reading can occur, it should be very easy to accept that literature is quite recyclable. A story can be read by a very young reader and understood in one way, while the same story can be read by a more advanced reader and understood in a very different way. As the middle school student is introduced to new complexities, he should also be exposed to different types of literature which allow for multilevel interpretations.

Teacher selection of reading material moves away from fairy tales, animal stories and myths where archetypal protagonists are flat and neutral, toward adventure stories, mysteries and biographies where narrative passages are replete with descriptions which reveal character motives, feelings and actions. An example of the possibilities for reusing or recycling stories is Steiner and Mueller's The Bear Who Wanted To Be A Bear (1976). This is a simple and beautifully illustrated story about a bear who is awakened from his nap by a construction crew building a huge factory. Emerging from his den, the bear is forced to become a factory machine operator. Personnel managers and executives do not listen to his plea, *" 'Excuse me,' the bear said politely, 'but I am a bear.' "* Unable to convince them of this, the bear is required to prove he is really a bear. He is forced to visit a circus and a zoo where other bears must confirm his true identity. But none of these environments are familiar and their inhabitants do not recognize the bear.

Compelled to return to the factory complex, the bear shaves and then dons overalls. He cannot conform to the working standards and is fired from his job for being a "lazybones." He trudges off into the surrounding wilderness and as the snow begins to fall once again in the woods *"the bear senses that he's forgotten something very important."*

Finally he remembers. The last picture in the book is a snow-covered den in front of which are fresh footprints and abandoned overalls.

For the adult or high school reader, twentieth century sensibilities are pricked, concerns for dehumanizing industrialization—its concurrent anxieties, disorientation, loss of personal identity, victimization and cancelled freedoms—may come to mind. For a middle school reader it might be a funny story with a play on appearances and realities, or it may be a personally significant story in which the reader identifies with the misunderstood bear. For a younger reader it can be a story about mean men and a very kind and patient bear, or perhaps even a sad story about losing one's home.

The levels of literary competence which determine the reading of the work can range from understanding of basic plot elements within the text, to identifying archetypal characters and themes, to comparing this story to other situations or stories either previously experienced or read.

SOME SPECIFIC LITERARY STRUCTURES

A structural approach attempts to identify a hierarchy of elements in literature so that reading and all learning experiences *"are attaching themselves to one another, and forming a larger pattern"* (Frye, 1972, p. 4). A fundamental element in the hierarchy of literary structures is the story contour or form as a whole; that is, its plot.

Plot is simply defined as sequenced actions taken from the events in a story. For the teacher, plot diagraming can be used to show that actions of a story are meaningfully linked in a progression that moves to an important point and then to some kind of resolution.

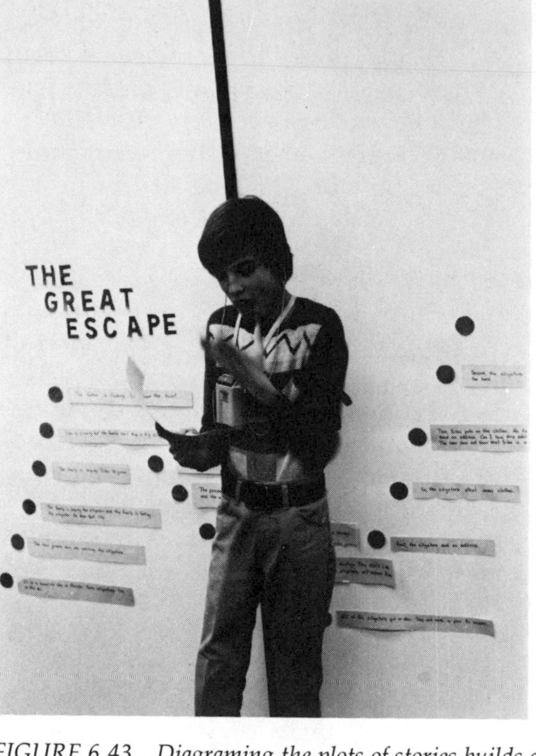

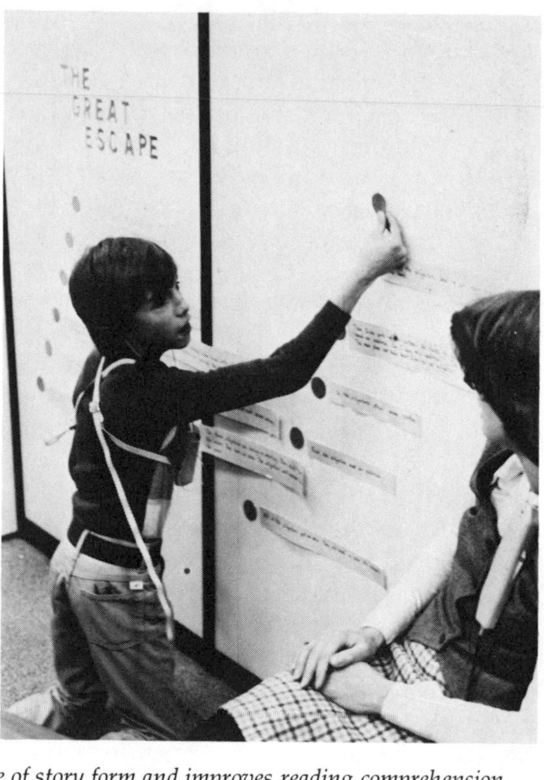

FIGURE 6.43 Diagraming the plots of stories builds a sense of story form and improves reading comprehension.

Many students never appreciate the structure of a story and many do not even feel the necessity to bring a story to a reasonable conclusion. Within the collection of troll stories discussed in the preceding section, there is a common type of plot progression that moves from posing a problem or conflict, through a series of well-defined events, and finally to a resolution. By mapping the action and iconically representing (or diagraming) it, similarities and differences in structure between one story and another can be effectively approached in class. *(FIGURE 6.43)* Diagraming the story structure can also facilitate the transfer of information; the reader can compare and contrast stories.

Having students predict the action of a story given the conflict or the first actions of a major character is a way to work on plot completion and to develop the skill of prediction in the reader. Each reader can complete the story or supply the necessary events as he or she imagines them and these various resolutions can then be used to rewrite the story as the students see it. This exercise gives students more confidence in their expressive language and more respect for their own creative potential.

When first approaching the task of plot completion, young readers tend to see stories as random collections of events related only by a constant set of characters who participate in these events. With a growing exposure to structure in stories, such as Stone Soup (McGovern, 1968) where an initial event reoccurs in a modified form and a final ironic event resolves the additive action, the child's response to similar additive story structure becomes more plausible.

Stone Soup is a classic tale in which a nameless young man comes to the home of an old woman and asks for something to eat.

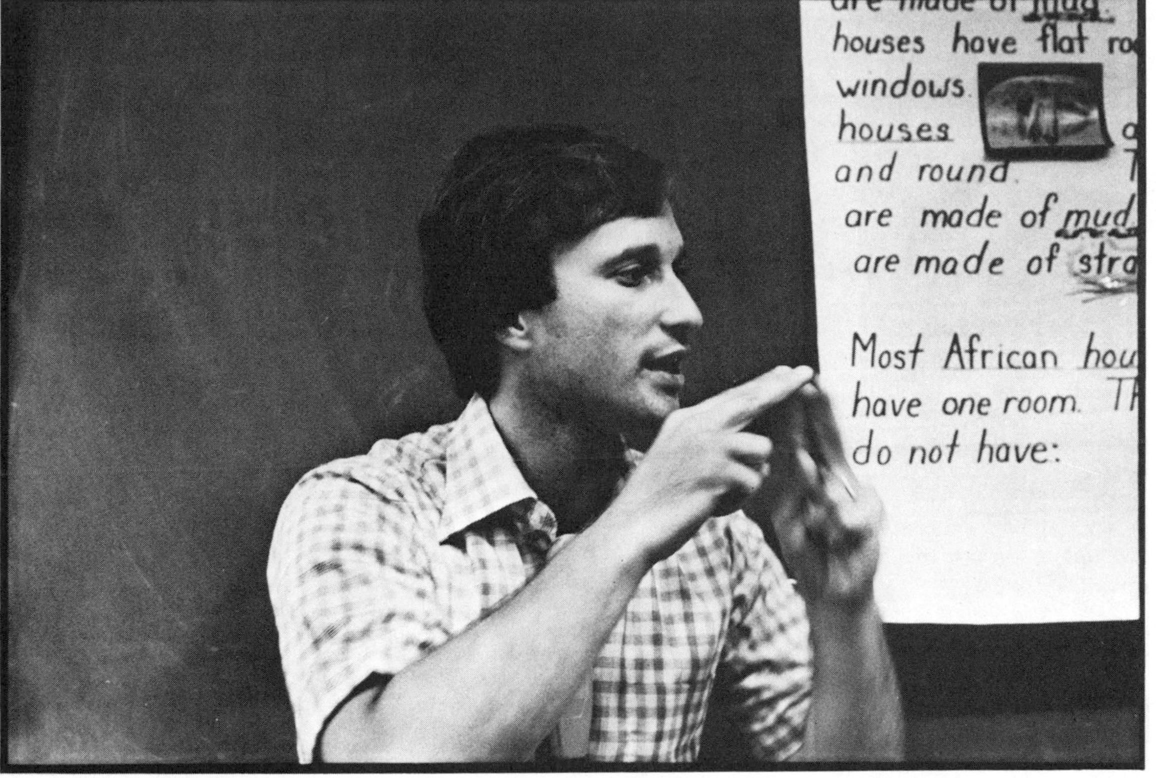
houses have flat
windows.
houses
and round.
are made of mud
are made of
Most African
have one room.
do not have:

FIGURE 6.44

Though the greedy woman claims she has no food to offer, the beggar convinces her that he can make soup from just one stone. Once a kettle is secured, the young man tricks the woman into adding a variety of ingredients to the boiling mixture. As the beggar eats the delicious soup, the woman is amazed at how much good could come from a single stone. If the young reader can learn to rely on his reading ability–his understanding of the structure of events in a story–then an over-dependence on particular reading skills which come slowly for the hearing-impaired reader (decoding, word recognition, complex linguistic structures) can be avoided.

Because story structures soon move away from simple event-oriented plots, the middle school reader must develop reading abilities which allow him to use both explicit and implicit information. If he is to comprehend attributes of characters and the actions which might motivate or determine the action of a story, if he is to qualify his responses to the characters and their acts by selecting only relevant or focal attributes, and if he is to use his own judgments to learn from a story, then his reading skills must include the cognitive processes of categorizing, labeling and subordinating, as well as the linguistic forms which explicitly code these processes.

Reader response to literary structure can be an index of cognitive status and reading competence. For example, the experience of a middle school class with Stone Soup indicated that the students' levels of understanding extended beyond an event orientation to more advanced comprehension of the attributes of the story's characters. This story, with its archetypal wanderer, greedy old woman and repetitive structure, may be read on a very elementary level. However, the plot constructions of a middle school class based

Today we put on our coats
and went outside. We were
playing ball and broke the
window. The teacher got mad.

Her voice growled fiercely. Her
face was all wrinkled up and got
very red. She put her hands on
her hips and she tapped her
foot quickly.

FIGURE 6.45 The contrast between narrative and descriptive language can be presented in the same context.

A Riddle.

Silas can't see
anything.

It is dark and murky.

His feet feel sticky
like he is walking
in mud.

WHERE IS SILAS?

FIGURE 6.46 Guessing by attributes

on this story indicated a movement into causally based perceptions of events and their sequencing. The characters and corresponding attributes determine the story's rising structure. Because the students recognized the beggar as truly clever and the old woman as gullible and foolish, they could predict and anticipate further events by using their understanding of what clever people and silly people usually do.

In class discussion, when children over use their understanding of attribute, the teacher is forced to redirect focus back to the relevant events of the story. *(FIGURE 6.44)* For example, children may retell a story with highly embellished actual or possible details of events or characters. Their diversions into personalized descriptions often become the occasion for class "rap-time," and though discussions are lively and enjoyable, the teacher is constantly aware of the need to bring the class back on target.

Refocusing a child's observations can be encouraged by designing materials that contain a narrative passage followed by a description of the event or character. *(FIGURE 6.45)* This structural pattern is similar to the topic/comment structure which organizes a single sentence. The entire narrative passage can become the topic and the succeeding description can be seen as a comment on the actions or characters.

This pattern of topic/comment or narration/description is often deleted when teachers rewrite materials for hearing-impaired students. If the intent of a chart or story is to encourage an awareness of description, the sequencing of events can become secondary to the class' dramatizations of expressions or figurative language. It is also possible to provide a description using the attributes of an event and to have the students guess what the event was, thereby making a riddle game. *(FIGURE 6.46)*

Although descriptive passages have appeared in the myths, fairy tales and experience stories read earlier in school, it is at the stage of complexity that readers must begin actually relying on implicit information within descriptive passages. Descriptive language had been intitially included in chart stories for exposure purposes, but now the more complex structures which carry the descriptive information should be recognized and comprehended.

Description allows the reader to infer important qualities of characters and hence motivations. Much of the descriptive data can be explicitly stated within a sentence containing, for example, a relative clause or an adverbial. However, the reader must also learn to critically sample, evaluate and subordinate one bit of descriptive information to another if the implicit message is to be understood. For example, in the sentence,

> The Queen was beautiful but wicked.

the focal attribute is the queen's wickedness; that is, despite the fact that the queen was beautiful, she was evil. Part of the selective process whereby some details are foregrounded and others are not will depend on the reader's active ability to anticipate textual information as well as understand different types of syntactic coordination.

Structures within science fiction stories and mysteries require both a sense of anticipation and prediction. In a mystery story or a story with a twist at the end, many of the details explicitly revealed by the author do not supply sufficient data to solve the riddle of the murder or mystery. Attending to the relevant descriptive details is an indispensable tool if a reader is to be truly involved in the unfolding of a plot or mystery. By recognizing the function of various types of descriptive structures (imparting of details, giving definitions, setting tone or mood, or delineating character traits), the more advanced reader can also learn to adjust his reading strategies to the task at hand.

Details are critical in certain textual passages, while in others they need not be given equivalent attention. At times one must look for descriptions which define if one is to understand an unfamiliar concept or imaginary character.

> *The trolls who had ribbons pinned to their knots were the highest of the high.*

And still in other instances, descriptions must be recognized as vehicles for conveying the tone or mood of a story.

> The water rat was restless, and he did not exactly know why. To all appearance, the summer's pomp was still at its fullest height, and although in the tilled acres green had given way to gold, though rowans were reddening, and the woods were dashed here and there with a tawny fierceness, yet light and warmth and colour were still present in undiminished measure, clean of any chilly premonitions of the passing year" (Grahame, 1969, p. 146).

It is very important that teachers, through contrastive exposure to the varying functions of descriptive structures, prevent the reading process from becoming a nonselective one in which all descriptive information is given equal weight by the reader. A skilled reader learns to discard details in descriptions that are not vital or relevant to the context in which they occur or to the over-all purpose of the reading.

Because the function of descriptive passages is not necessarily to convey action or plot movement, designing questions which assess the readers' understanding of these textual structures becomes very difficult. For example, in a rewritten passage based on Mayer's A Special Trick (1976),

> Now Elroy was alone in the room.
> Carefully he swept under the table. On the table Elroy saw black boxes and black hats.
> Did that hat move?
> Did that box talk?

a common questioning technique would be to ask,

> "Where did Elroy sweep?"

The child who is unable to answer such a question may be diagnosed as having difficulties with language structures involving prepositions or *wh* pro-forms. However, because the question is requiring the child to attend to an element in the descriptive passage which is not conceptually salient or relevant (the table), it is actually the question rather than the child's response which is inappropriate. It is important, then, for the teacher to consider what information is critical in and representative of the child's understanding of descriptive structures.

In addition to structures of narration and description, the reader must also come to appreciate structures such as **theme.** Pure linguistic comprehension is not sufficient in understanding the universal themes which structure the many forms of reading material he will encounter. The reader needs to know that a character setting out on a journey will meet with obstacles and that these obstacles can be overcome. This story theme structures the *romance.* The reader must know that good people can have flaws which ruin them or that good people are sometimes destroyed by others. This theme dominates the *tragedy.* And the reader must accept that people can be pawns in situations far beyond their control; this is *comedy* or *irony.* These understandings make the ordering of one's own experiences through literature possible.

Narration/description format, plot contours and themes can all be seen as **intertextual** literary structures and can be recognized as organizing units which appear and reappear across a wide range of story forms. Teachers of English should be aware that frequent exposure to these recursive elements will be required before they can become truly functional as organizing units for the reader. Bombarding the reader with all types of stories, even while controlling for vocabulary and syntax, will not necessarily produce readers who can develop meaningful categories for stories. The responsibility of selecting and synthesizing materials so that specific literary structures are highlighted belongs to the teacher.

There are, in addition to intertextual structures, those which organize elements within a single work. These **intratextual** structures allow the reading process to become an active performance whereby the reader can organize pervious textual information occurring in the story to accommodate new information. As Parker (1969) notes,

"Reading prose fiction then is a process of relating the hints held within the mystery of the story to the aspects of story already known. It is a process of assimilating meaning to a developing conception of story, and of revising that conception to accommodate new meanings. In this process the complex elements of story are related by a wholistic image"(p. 100).

Research shows that efficient readers can predict events and structures on many levels of processing: syntactic, lexical, narrative. Prediction in reading, claims F. Smith (1970), *"involves the reduction of uncertainty through the elimination of unlikely alternatives* (p. 305)." By capitalizing on the syntactic as well as semantic redundancies which characterize written language, the reader can learn to predict by discarding unlikely possibilities for the meaning of a word or passage. Prediction, then, is a feed-forward system which can be activated on many levels. Just as clues can function to signal a fantasy theme on the intertextual level, so are there cues or clues hidden within a text which will allow for more accurate predictions on an intratextual level.

A brief look at the traditional Grimm's fairy tale "Snow White" may be used to illustrate structures which function as clues to the reader. For instance, when the huntsman takes Snow White into the woods and is required by the wicked Queen to cut out Snow White's lung and liver and return them to the Queen, the young reader must recognize that the lung and liver will represent Snow White's death. The lung and liver must function as clues to the slaying of the young girl if the huntsman's act is not to be seen as something grotesque and unmotivated. If the reader cannot anticipate what the huntsman does with the lungs and liver of the bear, which he has slain in the place of Snow White, the reader might be led astray by becoming preoccupied with the huntsman's brutal act. The student who focuses on the act itself without understanding the motivation behind it will seriously misread the text. Since the plot will depend on the Queen thinking that Snow White is dead, this clue must be established early in the story.

Snow White runs deep into the woods and comes upon the cottage of the seven dwarfs. An iconic description (seven knives, seven forks, etc.) can function as a clue to the reader. Upon their return home, the dwarfs ponder over the little hollows found in their beds where Snow White had tried unsuccessfully to make herself comfortable. Each dwarf knows that "Someone has been sleeping in my bed." However, the reader knows a bit more.

This same type of active reading plays a strong part in the child's appreciation of the dwarfs' warning to Snow White cautioning her about the wicked Queen. Drawn by her own vanity, the Queen approaches the looking glass asking

> "Mirror, mirror on the wall, who is the fairest in all the land?"

The mirror proclaims that it is Snow White.

As the story unfolds, the Queen's question itself takes on a greater significance. Not only must the reader anticipate the mirror's answer but he must also see the causal relationship at work between the Queen approaching the mirror and her coming away determined once again to destroy Snow White. This scene reoccurs twice more within the story. Through its repetition it becomes an intratextual clue which triggers and reinforces a reader's predictions.

The task of the teacher in rewriting material is to be conscious of such intratextual elements or clues that the reader can use to develop sophisticated reading abilities. While simplifying literary texts to suit the language level of the hearing-impaired student may be necessary, texts can also be made accessible if the contextual and semantic cues which structure the story are preserved and if readers develop the strategies which make use of these structures. In much of the new relevancy literature with a high-interest, low-reading level, many structural elements are eliminated. While the intent of much of this realistic literature is to encourage non-readers to read, its simplified format can in fact make the reading task more difficult.

The need to find literature which is syntactically less complex may have serious consequences, for it may inhibit a major potential of literature within a curriculum; that is, helping readers make reasoned judgments. If the student is not only to learn to read but also to learn from reading, the literature he encounters as an introduction to complexity must be in tune with his cognitive, psychological and social development.

SUGGESTED READINGS

READING AND LITERATURE

Egoff, S., Stubbs, G., & Ashley, L. *Only connect.* Toronto: Oxford University Press, 1969.
Frye, N. *On teaching literature.* New York: Harcourt, Brace, & Jovanovich, 1972.
Smith, F. *Understanding reading.* New York: Holt, Rinehart, & Winston, 1971.
Stewig, J. *Read to write.* New York: Hawthorne Books, Inc., 1975.

LINGUISTICS

Chomsky, C. *The acquisition of syntax in children from 5 to 10.* Cambridge, MA: M.I.T. Press, 1969.
Lester, M. *Readings in applied transformational grammar.* New York: Holt, Rinehart, & Winston, 1970.
Limber, J. The genesis of complex sentences. In T. Moore (Ed.), *Cognition and the acquisition of language.* New York: Academic Press, 1973.
Reibel, D., & Schane, S. *Modern studies in English: Readings in transformational grammar.* Englewood Cliffs, N.J.: Prentice Hall, 1969.

ACKNOWLEDGMENTS

FIGURES

Page 92 *Figure 6.39,* Page 93 *Figure 6.40* Courtesy of Lois Fain, Rhode Island School for the Deaf.
Page 95 *Figure 6.41* From unit prepared by John Plante, Rhode Island School for the Deaf.
Page 96 From units prepared by Marilyn Cooney, Donna Spang, and Mary Weiner, Rhode Island School for the Deaf.
Page 97 From unit prepared by Peggy Vale, Rhode Island School for the Deaf.
Page 98 *Figure 6.42* From unit prepared by Judy Tartaglia, Rhode Island School for the Deaf.
Page 102 *Figure 6.43* From unit prepared by Mary Jane Stumpe, Rhode Island School for the Deaf.
Page 103 *Figure 6.44* Photograph courtesy of Ira Garber.

Chapter 7

The Expansion of Complexity

To meet the changing demands created by cognitive growth, an expanding social environment and a broadening of content matter, the adolescent student must develop a more efficient use of complex linguistic structures and an increased competence and flexibility in reading. Basal readers, which are of less interest and relevance to the student approaching adolescence, are replaced by individualized projects such as letter writing and journal keeping. Newspaper articles and information-filled textbooks may also become prominent parts of the classroom experience. In addition, students can be asked to use the library and other resource areas.

Yet one cannot assume that sheer practice in reading skills or continued exposure to complex linguistic structures alone will enable the student to successfully meet these new challenges. Along with the growing and changing needs of students entering junior high school, there are the greater expectations of the teachers themselves, as well as a marked change in the teaching environment.

Unlike the earlier school years, methods of instruction are no longer restricted by the kinds of skills and content to be mastered. Generally, students are now more comfortable with less structured learning situations and are expected to be more independent in deciding how time is spent and what methods of inquiry they will use to solve particular problems. This is especially important in reading. Whether in a classroom reading area or a school library, students begin using unstructured time more as an extension of their own interests as well as to meet the demands of their school work. Student involvement in the selection of reading materials will be tempered, first by their cognitive and social readiness and secondly by the linguistic complexity of the materials.

The new types of literature now being chosen by students bring with them more complex and stylized language constructions and transformations. Similarly, the increasing complexity of the cognitive and informational nature of textbooks is reflected in more complex language. If newspapers and magazines are referred to, there is the use of deletions, transformations for style purposes and more idiomatic language.

All of this contributes to the students' need to expand their language and reading abilities. Continued organized exposure to the widening array of complex linguistic and literary structures can build upon the basic categories that the child has already established. Thus, for students moving into this developmental stage, the teacher can set as goals the mastery–the understanding and use–of several identifiable, complex linguistic and literary forms.

Complex Linguistic Structures

The three linguistic processes discussed in this section, **complementation, nominalization,** and **deletion,** assume competency in the processes described in Chapter 6; relativization, conjunction, and movement transformations that are sentence internal (passive) or move clauses (adverbial movement). The particular order in which these structures and processes appear is not the issue here but rather the students' cognitive and linguistic readiness to deal with them. The readiness of the students to move to this more complex level can be measured by their ability to comprehend and use the complex syntactic structures covered in the preceding stage: relative clauses, conjunctions and adverbials.

The new structures presented here are only a small sampling of the kinds of complex language constructions that students will meet as their reading and communicative competencies expand. But once mastered, these structures become new tools for generalizing about the form and content of new information encountered in classwork and especially in reading materials.

Although the next level in the language developmental hierarchy is difficult to define specifically, there appears a significant jump from the structures discussed in Chapter 6 to the kinds of complex structures discussed here. The difference, however, seems to relate to several areas: increased use of whole clauses as the subject or object of a sentence, the morphological changes related to syntactic movement, increased sentence length, and the increased use of deletions and other embedding transformations that make the use of a whole sentence as a subject or object less cumbersome. Understanding and being aware of these linguistic factors is an important step in effective teaching at this level.

NOUN PHRASE COMPLEMENTATION

"One problem with noun phrase complementation, nominalization, and any other process embedding one sentence structure inside another, is that, as in this sentence which you are presently reading, it is all too easy, even with a firm determination to express important ideas, to get lost inside a complex sentence and either to say things you don't mean or to make grammatical errors which won't seem obvious upon first reading but which impedes comprehension" (Jacobs & Rosenbaum, 1971, p. 117).

Students who will make effective use of noun phrase complementation enter this stage having done previous work on noun phrases and embedding. Now the task is to put the two together. Students have already expanded noun phrases (NPs) in their work on conjunctions, question work and in the expansion of noun phrases by adding adjectives or possessives. They have also had experience with syntactic embeddings in their work on relative and adverbial clauses. But these have been cases, semantically, where a sentence describes or places another sentence in time or space. Noun phrase complementation, on the other hand, is where a whole sentence acts like a noun phrase and it serves as either the semantic subject or object of the verb.

In fact, students have had some exposure to this structure in the direct discourse so frequently found in basal readers:

The wolf said, *"I will eat Little Red Riding Hood."*

Although the quoted sentence is a complete sentence, it is also functioning as the object of the verb *said*. The quoted sentence could then be analyzed as NP_2 of sentence pattern two.

In indirect speech, the same sentence would become:

The wolf said *that he would eat Little Red Riding Hood.*

The analysis of this sentence is similar to the one in direct speech but it has been transformed into indirect discourse by an embedding transformation. Added is the complementizer *that* and changed is the pronoun from *I* to *he* and the verb from *will* to *would*. The embedded sentence (the triangle in *FIGURE 7.47*), though harder to recognize, is also functioning as an object noun phrase. Noun phrase complements have been encountered as early as the lower school years, especially in the so-called infinitive complement *(FIGURE 7.48)*. These structures are very similar in underlying structure to that in *FIGURE 7.47*. In both examples of noun phrase complements, the child must recognize the whole sentence (represented by the triangle in the

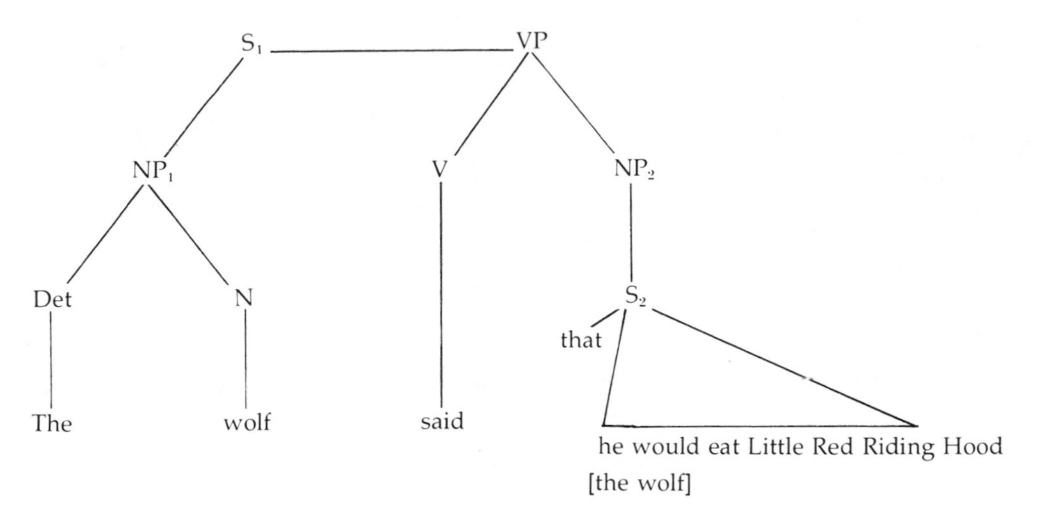

FIGURE 7.47 Tree diagram

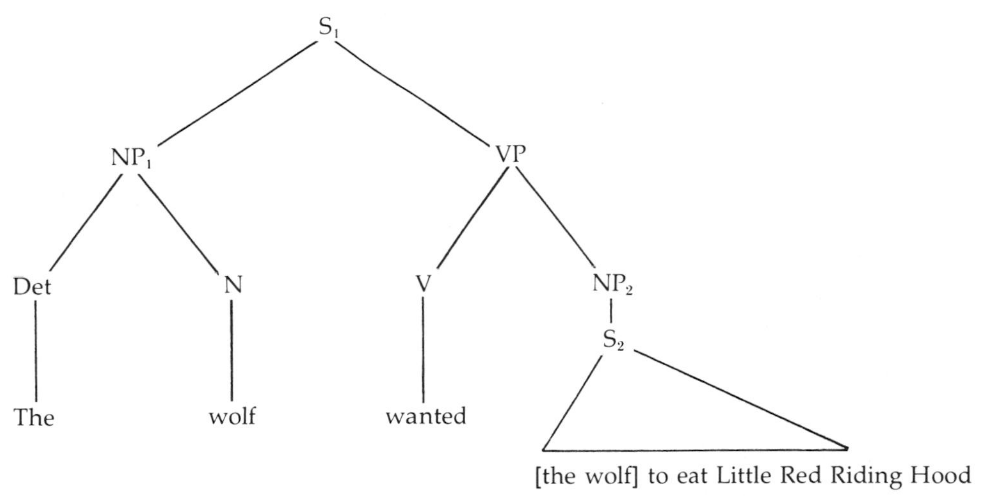

FIGURE 7.48 Tree diagram for infinitive complement sentence

tree diagrams) as an object noun phrase of the larger sentence. Once the student has internalized that sentences can function as simple noun phrases, then more advanced types of complementation can be acquired.

Additional difficulties experienced by students with this type of structure involve changes in stress and intonational contours that occur when declaratives, interrogatives or imperatives are embedded into larger sentences. For example, one student may ask another in the class, "What do you like?" This sentence has a marked question intonation pattern. If another student is asked to restate the question, the sentence becomes "John asked what you like." The *what* in the sentence is unstressed and attention to stress changes in embedded sentences should be included as part of the speech program in the classroom. Similarly, if one student says "Sit down!" and another student is asked to repeat this indirectly, the sentence is transformed to "John said to sit down." These sentences also have markedly different intonational contours and, in addition, the embedded sentence contains the noun phrase complement, *to sit down*.

This syntactic process is common in social interaction, especially in the reporting of what another has said. Thus, classroom work on this particular structure can address three general areas that are problematical for hearing-impaired students at this level:

1. **Syntactic Development:** The ability to expand the NP_2 position and use full sentences in that position. This includes the ability to comprehend embedded sentences despite the morphological or intonational changes that have taken place in the embedding process.

2. **Speech:** The development of appropriate intonational contours for embedded sentence types (imperatives, interrogatives and declaratives).

3. **Affective Growth:** The ability to accurately report what another has said without syntactic or semantic distortion. This includes

Carter's strategy for cities outlined

TUCSON, Ariz. (UPI) — HUD Secretary Patricia Harris today promised the nation's mayors a new urban strategy under the Carter administration, but she warned that federal money may be withheld from cities failing to reduce the "isolation" of the poor.

Mrs. Harris, in remarks prepared for delivery to the U.S. Conference of Mayors, said the administration strategy involves "shoring up" economic and tax bases of distressed cities, conserving inner-city neighborhoods and providing fair housing opportunities for low-income families in cities and suburbs.

She also said the role of mayors will be strengthened in future planning.

But Mrs. Harris warned that cities failing to adhere to equal opportunity provisions of the Housing Assistance Plan could lose federal block grants.

She said she will allocate up to 20,000 units of Section 8 rehabilitated housing to aid cities in neighborhood conservation efforts.

Mrs. Harris said President Carter is committed to ending "the politics of fear" in the cities, saying he "broke the back" of the politics of racial confrontation.

"The lessons of the past," she said, "should remind us that all of our plans, all our programs and all our good intentions can be violently swept aside by forces which are easy to trigger but very difficult to control."

FIGURE 7.49 Noun phrase complements beginning with the word that are common occurrences in newspaper articles.

the ability to perceive when another person is reporting indirectly.

The reporting function of noun phrase complements brings us to another frequent use of this structure. Noun phrase complements are among the most commonly occurring structures in newspapers and need to be understood if the student is to use this type of material in class or, ultimately, to use it independently. *(FIGURE 7.49)* In many reports, a transformation called topicalization is applied to help focus the reader's attention on the complement sentence. This transformation moves the complement to the front of the sentence. Thus, the sentence

The White House announced today that the President will attend a conference in Geneva,

becomes a different sentence when topicalization is applied.

The President will attend a conference in Geneva, the White House announced today,

is different from the nominalizations where

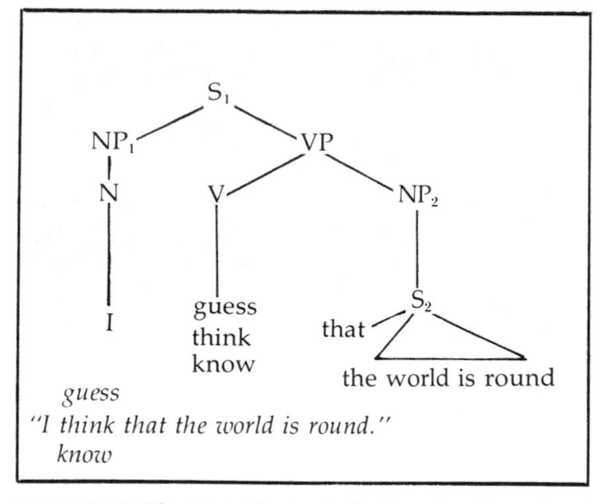

FIGURE 7.50 Tree diagram of noun phrase complement after verbs of mental state.

the noun phrase actually functions as the subject of the sentence. In addition to understanding change in emphasis in sentences to which topicalization has been applied, students should be able to read these with the appropriate intonational contour.

Using noun phrase complements correctly also requires understanding of the semantic differences in the verbs that take object complements. Some of these verbs, such as *think, guess, know* and *believe,* have subtle differences in meaning which convey different things about the speaker's state of mind. In addition, these verbs all take syntactic complements beginning with the complementizer *that*. The underlying structure of these sentences is illustrated in *FIGURE 7.50.*

Activities that involve guessing at a number or the estimation of distance, weight or height are good ways of introducing students to different verb types and meanings. If the task is to estimate the distance to a classroom door, the students' guesses can be put into the appropriate linguistic form.

Bill guessed *that the door is ten feet away.*
Maria estimated *that the door was four feet away.*

This kind of exercise may also produce other useful information for the teacher about how

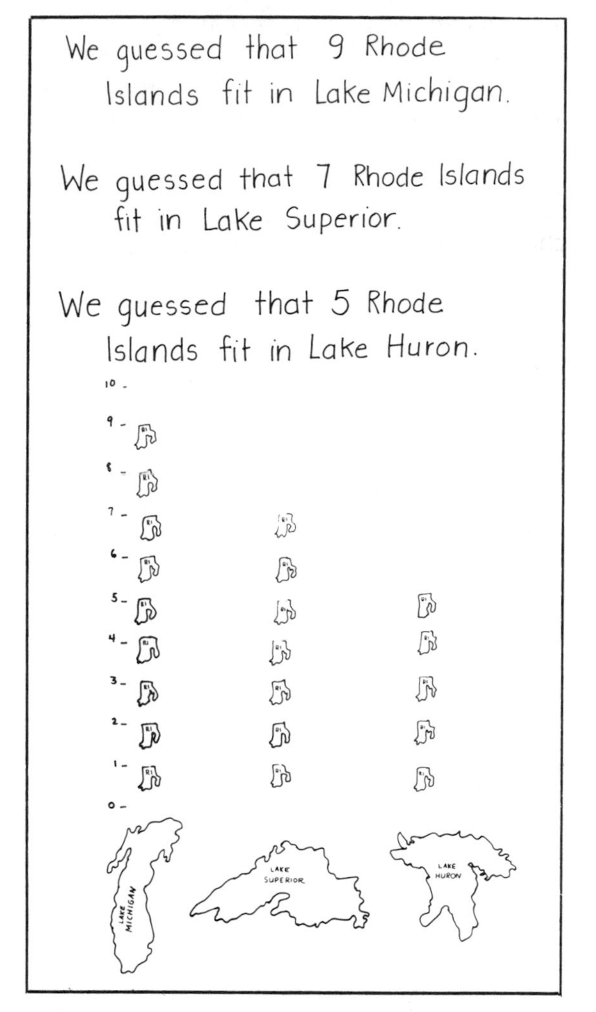
We guessed that 9 Rhode Islands fit in Lake Michigan.
We guessed that 7 Rhode Islands fit in Lake Superior.
We guessed that 5 Rhode Islands fit in Lake Huron.
10
9
8
7
6
5
4
3
2
1
0
LAKE MICHIGAN
LAKE SUPERIOR
LAKE HURON

FIGURE 7.51 An activity within the Paddle-to-the-Sea unit discussed in Chapter 2 required the children to estimate the area of three great lakes in relation to the area of Rhode Island.

well a particular student can estimate or conjecture and how comfortable or confident a student is with that skill. If desired, this activity can be continued by actually measuring the distance to the door and then calculating the differences between the actual measurement and the students' estimations. This might help the student whose estimate is far off the mark to modify his estimate, especially if the results are recorded iconically as well as symbolically. *(FIGURE 7.51)*

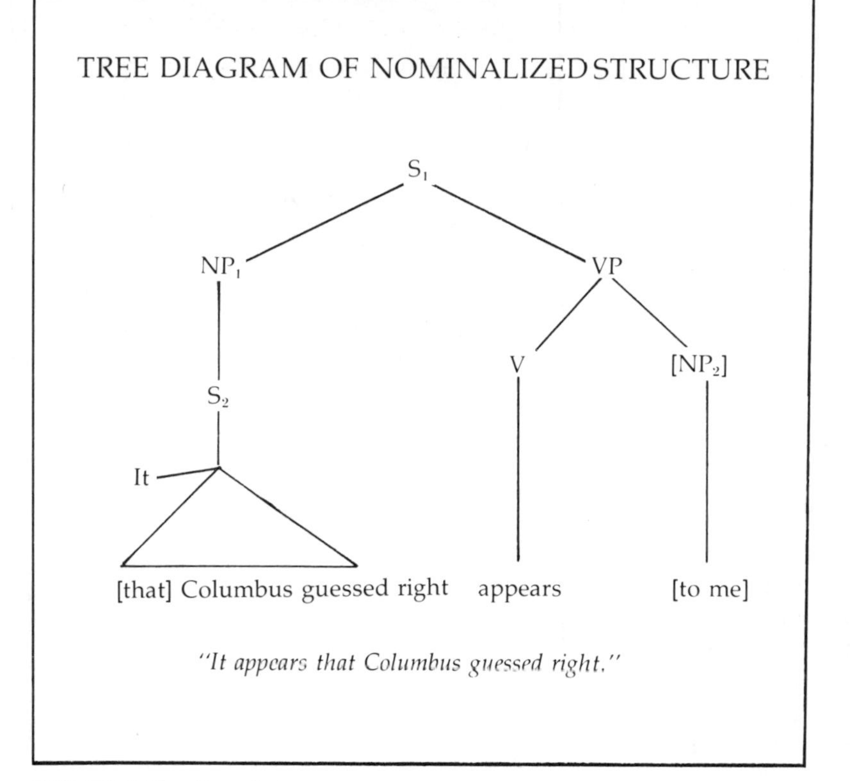

FIGURE 7.52 Tree diagram

Hypothesizing, as in the preceding example, is an important skill in many areas. Therefore, the job of helping the students acquire the linguistic tools to express this cognitive ability is not just the English teacher's, but one that concerns all teachers.

Opinion making, an important part of the adolescent's affective growth and functioning, can also be a productive source for work on noun phrase complements. As so many people have noted, hearing-impaired students tend to be very categorical in their opinion-making process. This may result from a lack of critical thinking experiences at an earlier level and often is perpetuated by the student's unfamiliarity with the language structures and verb types needed to express ambiguous or noncategorical thinking.

Verbs of personal belief, such as *I believe, I guess, I suppose,* are often all blended into *I know* by the hearing-impaired student and thus the relationship between the complement and the meaning of the verb is lost. Faced with a sentence like,

> Columbus *believed* [that the earth was flat] when he sailed,

the hearing-impaired student who misinterprets *believed* is likely to respond with,

> Columbus stupid.

If, however, the student understands that beliefs can be educated guesses as opposed to the sense of having complete faith in, then Columbus' belief (the bracketed complement) is easier to accept and understand. Work on verbs of personal belief and the complements they take is one way of integrating conceptual and linguistic considerations in teaching.

A final type of complement to be considered leads to the next section on nominalizations. Very often students encounter sentences like,

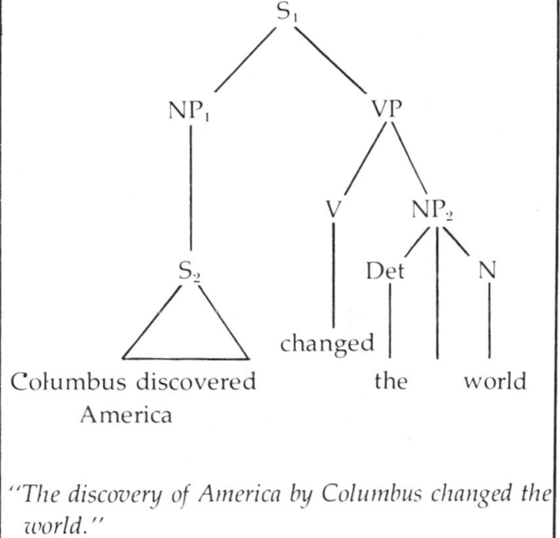

FIGURE 7.53 Tree diagram of the deep structure before transformations have applied for the sentence.

It appears that Columbus guessed right.

In this sentence the *it* is not really the subject of the sentence; rather the subject is the *that* clause. The deep structure of this sentence is illustrated in *FIGURE 7.52.*

Understanding that a whole sentence can semantically serve as a subject even when it is in the object position is a difficult task. But if this kind of structure can be mastered, the common occurrence of nominalized sentences in subject position can also be understood and productively used.

NOMINALIZATION

Nominalization requires the students to possess cognitive and linguistic skills that enable them to interpret entire sentences as subjects or objects. In addition, it requires the stu-

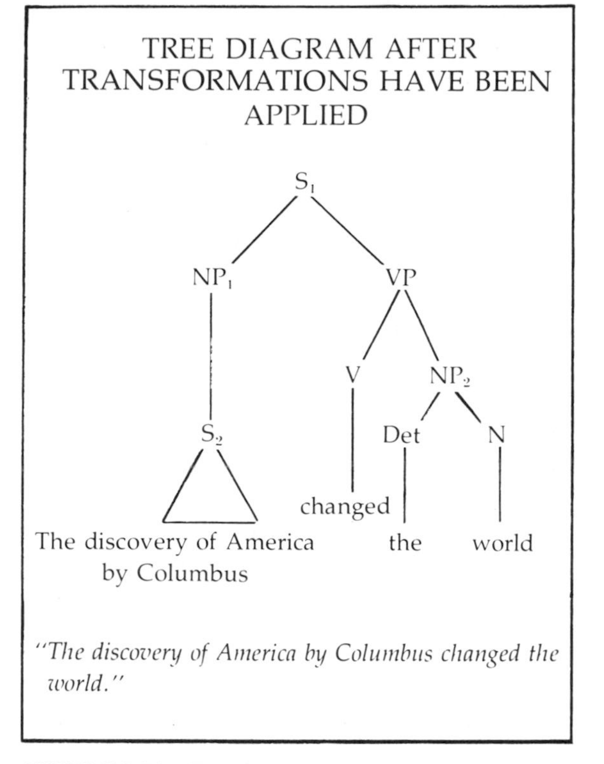

FIGURE 7.54 Tree diagram of derived structure after transformations have applied.

dents to interpret sentences from which the nominalization process has seemingly removed the verb and which may have been otherwise transformed (passivized, for example). Very often this happens in subject position, as is the case of this sentence from a social studies lesson:

> The discovery of America by Columbus changed the world.

This sentence comes from the deep structure diagramed in *FIGURE 7.53.*

To arrive at the surface sentence, the passive transformation has been applied and the main verb of the embedded sentence is no longer apparent. After these transformations, the derived structure looks like that in *FIGURE 7.54*. The nominalization process allows the underlying verb of the original embedded sentence, *discover,* to become the semantic focus of the sentence, as *discovery.*

There are several ways to work through sentences in class with the students' previously established skills in kernelization and sentence pattern identification coming into play. Breaking the sentence down first into kernels allows the students to begin by analyzing these sentence parts. By identifying the embedded sentence *"Columbus discovered America"* as a pattern two, the students can find the verb *discover* and relate it to the nominalized form, *discovery*. Rather than doing contrasting morphology work by list or out of context, pairs like *discover/discovery* can be done in the context of work on syntax. If the sentences are from a social studies lesson, the conceptual background is there as well.

After working with the embedded sentence in the NP_1 position, the matrix sentence can be identified by sentence pattern. The above example is a sentence pattern two and students can see the whole sentence made up of two little sentence pattern twos. The principle of little sentences making big sentences is reinforced and applied in this way.

Carter's strategy for cities outlined

TUCSON, Ariz. (UPI) — HUD Secretary Patricia Harris today promised the nation's mayors a new urban strategy under the Carter administration, but she warned that federal money may be withheld from cities failing to reduce the "isolation" of the poor.

Mrs. Harris, in remarks prepared for delivery to the U.S. Conference of Mayors, said the administration strategy involves "shoring up" economic and tax bases of distressed cities, conserving inner-city neighborhoods and providing fair housing opportunities for low-income families in cities and suburbs.

She also said the role of mayors will be strengthened in future planning.

She said she will allocate up to 20,000 units of Section 8 rehabilitated housing to aid cities in neighborhood conservation efforts.

Mrs. Harris said President Carter is committed to ending "the politics of fear" in the cities, saying he "broke the back" of the politics of racial confrontation.

"The lessons of the past," she said, "should remind us that all of our plans, all our programs and all our good intentions can be violently swept aside by forces which are easy to trigger but very difficult to control."

FIGURE 7.55 Newspaper articles often have many deletions that make familiar structures difficult to recognize.

DELETION

Linguistic complexity results from the nature of the structures themselves as well as from the functions that the structures serve. For example, newspaper language is often very complex because of the need to say a great deal in a limited space. This causes numerous syntactic deletions. (*FIGURE 7.55*)

(a) John believed he would win the prize.
(b) John believed that he would win the prize.

The above sentence (a) has deleted the complementizer *that*. Students who have had experience with the deletion of relative pronouns find the process itself easier to recognize. To effectively process such sentences the student needs to know that a deletion has taken place, that the embedded sentence is still a sentence, what has been deleted, and that this kind of deletion does not change the meaning of the sentence. The student cannot be functioning only at a surface structure level, and efficient language processing at this stage requires the comprehension and use of an underlying (deep) structure.

This section has explored some areas of syntactic complexity that are troublesome for hearing-impaired students but must be dealt with if the student is to grow educationally. When working on these structures, the teacher should focus on the processes that underlie particular transformations, not the rote operation of each. In addition, the semantic function of whole sentences within other sentences should be emphasized. The relationship of these processes and structures to increased efficiency in reading, and the ability of the teacher to use these structures in a literature program, are discussed next.

Functions of Complex Linguistic Structures in Reading and Writing

As students begin learning more sophisticated strategies of organization–those that enhance both the efficiency of reading and hence the enjoyment of reading–the reading process itself becomes a channel for much more critical thought and learning.

Literature read critically carries the reader from the enactive (or in literature, dramatic) situation to the connotative or symbolic level. The emergence of the symbolic is dependent upon an entire network of reading skills and abilities. The systems of organization which make up these skills and abilities can range from extracting the main idea from a text, to recognition of narrative voice and intent, to meaningfully interpreting the most elaborate of metaphorical imagery.

If the functions of reading are to steadily broaden and refine the student's knowledge of the world, mastery of the complex linguistic structures discussed previously must be integrated with a mastery of complexities within the structure of literary forms as well. One must teach to both the reading of texts, which use these complex linguistic structures, and to those literary forms that demand similar processes and performances.

NARRATIVE VOICE

Reading material is most controlled at less complex levels, but with the increased use of textbooks, newspapers and work on research and report writing, more burden is placed on the student to select the critical data and make inferences which previously were a more overt function of the class situation and materials.

One of the most persistent difficulties for students is the use of the narrative voice and point of view. Who is speaking to whom in a text and why? Too often when we ask, "Why did the author write this story?," the response is, "Because it is a good story." There is very little understanding of sense of purpose in writing. One could probably trace this problem all the way back to the reader's inability to see some connection between dialogue and narrative discourse. Narrative, in a sense, can be seen as dialogue without quotation marks. However, the two people implicit in dialogue are not necessarily present in narrative discourse. A writer can be speaking to numerous types of audiences and can draw attention to or conceal his presence. The narrator can be obviously present, as in the first person voice of Paul Simon's "El Condor Pasa," *"I'd rather be a forest than a street,"* or the narrator can function omnisciently (third person) while seemingly absent, as in Tennyson's "The Eagle." (*FIGURE 7.56*) There are, of course, variations in the degree of narrator omniscience.

"THE EAGLE"

He clasps the crag with crooked hands;
Close to the sun in lonely lands,
Ringed with the azure world he stands.

The wrinkled sea beneath him crawls;
He watches from his mountain walls,
And like a thunderbolt he falls.

FIGURE 7.56

Both of these poems forcefully employ metaphors to carry their import (freedom, power), but the writer's techniques for manipulating the narrative voice also contribute to the reader's comprehension of the text. While one narrator is making a statement about his response to modern dehumanized life (Paul Simon's *"I'd rather be a forest than a street"*), the other is showing his reverence for something of nature. The potentials for language and communication are thus broadened by an appreciation of the personal statement made by the writer. By creating in

"DREAMS"

Hold fast to dreams
For if dreams die
Life is a broken-winged bird
That cannot fly.

Hold fast to dreams
For when dreams go
Life is a barren field
Frozen with snow.

"DREAM DEFERRED"

What happens to a dream deferred?
Does it dry up
like a raisin in the sun?
Or fester like a sore—
And then run?
Does it stink like rotten meat?
Or crust and sugar over—
like a syrupy sweet?

Maybe it just sags
like a heavy load.

Or does it explode?

FIGURE 7.57

the reader a sense of wonder in the majesty of the eagle, Tennyson permits us to appreciate not only nature, but the intent of the composer himself. Thus, each artist's creation affects our own perception of the world.

Too often while expanding their writing and reading competencies, students have not paid enough attention to elements of narrative discourse. The composing process in writing is limited to straight forward first or third person voiceless narration, and the student's reading development usually proceeds in the same way. For such readers, a good story or poem exists as an isolated entity, largely incapable of replication in their world and hence not truly an object of vicarious appreciation. It exists almost as an autonomous plot construction. In a spiraling conceptual curriculum accenting the development of man within an historical perspective, an important part of the student's understanding is that some situations are unique to certain people's experiences, and people's responses to their individual experiences are manifested in various ways.

Earlier in the curriculum, myths became examples of archetypal plots with morals. They should now also begin to reflect the teller's conceptions of his world's human condition. This requires the reader to be able to identify a narrator's voice and judge its reliability and intent. For example, the narrator of a legend from New Guinea may explain the growth of a garden by ascribing it to the moon's late night activities.

"Once a man came, planted a banana and a taro, and went home. The moon came up, saw this, planted the whole garden, and went back to its place" (McElhanon, 1974, p. 36).

The reader must realize that the narrator's description of the moon is a reflection of his particular culture's world view.

A meaningful introduction to the study of narrative voice is the juxtaposing of one voice to another, both speaking to the same theme. Thus we read Langston Hughes' "Dreams" and compare the narrator's point of view to that of the narrator in his "Dream Deferred." *(FIGURE 7.57)* Both voices speak about the essentiality of dreams, but to the first narrator the consequence of dreams lost is a withering life that becomes a "winged bird that cannot fly." For the second voice, a lost dream "explodes."

A reader may grasp the metaphoric or symbolic interpretation of the text, but a very strong part of what makes literature a vicarious experience–something which somehow orders the chaos of our lives–is diminished unless the reader knows which character is actually talking, what he is trying to express (meaning) and what this says about his philosophy, his audience and his topic (import).

Tremendous quantities of relevant literature must be used to provide the basis from which readers can independently compare, contrast and evaluate meaning and import. It is not sufficient to expose the reader to a narrative voice in a romance, a tragedy and a comedy and assume that readers will then independently grasp the voices of overstated melodrama, propaganda or irony. There is a danger in trying to teach by analogy when only a few examples are experienced. Reading two or three pieces on the same theme but with different types of narrators is not sufficient. Aside from the natural incubation period that a learner requires, the teacher's thematic grouping of material does not clarify the analogy. Narrators employ various styles of speaking and use different forms of text with which the student may not be familiar.

Stylistically, the monologue-type discourse becomes more apparent at this level of complexity. The majority of literature read by adolescent students is text containing a very visible or audible voice. This style pervades not only the best of the literature but the more mediocre of the new relevancy literature as well. Examples of the first type of literature are a young girl, new to a neighborhood, talking in the book, Jennifer, Hecate, Macbeth, William McKinley, and Me, Elizabeth (Konigsberg, 1967); or two high school students conversing in The Pigman (Zindel, 1968). The same first person narrative voice is found in the relevancy literature as well; for example, the voice of a young boy caught in the middle of his parents' divorce in the book, My Dad Lives in a Downtown Hotel (Mann, 1973).

The chief problem with the less successful texts is not their obvious intrusive narrator but their telling the reader too much instead of allowing the narrative to do the revealing:

"Henry, the elevator man, is always making jokes about me and Sheila. He thinks we like each other. The truth is, I can't stand her. She's a real know-it-all" (Blume, 1972, p. 43).

There is very little depth of perception on the part of some of these narrators and far too little successful use of critical writing. Thus the readers' performances are less complex.

POINT OF VIEW

Both teacher and student preparedness to deal with perspective or point of view usually proceeds on two levels; visually, seeing different things in different ways, and attitudinally, having different opinions concerning things. It is on the second broad attitudinal plane that the most difficulty is encountered. In this sense, point of view is simply evaluative and based on a person's opinions. In developing an awareness of who is talking, the readers should be encouraged to see characters and information in a less categorical way, allowing them to abstract actions from people and to objectify both the actions (or events) and the characters (or agents). This makes understanding of ambiguity and multiple interpretation possible.

The choice of materials as well as level of questioning and complexity of activities begin to draw attention to the techniques of narration in extended discourse. If texts are to promote more reasoned decision making and knowledgeable responses, then students need tools to interpret the subtle criteria which provide the basis for such judgments.

NARRATIVE AWARENESS THROUGH WRITING

As mentioned in the discussion of noun phrase complements, both diary and journal writing can help relate dialogue to narrative discourse and focus in on speaker/hearer relationships. These writing and reading forms are also used to encourage awareness of writer's perspective (narrator's voice) and to enhance the reader's comprehension.

The students are traditionally asked to keep journals for recording something per-

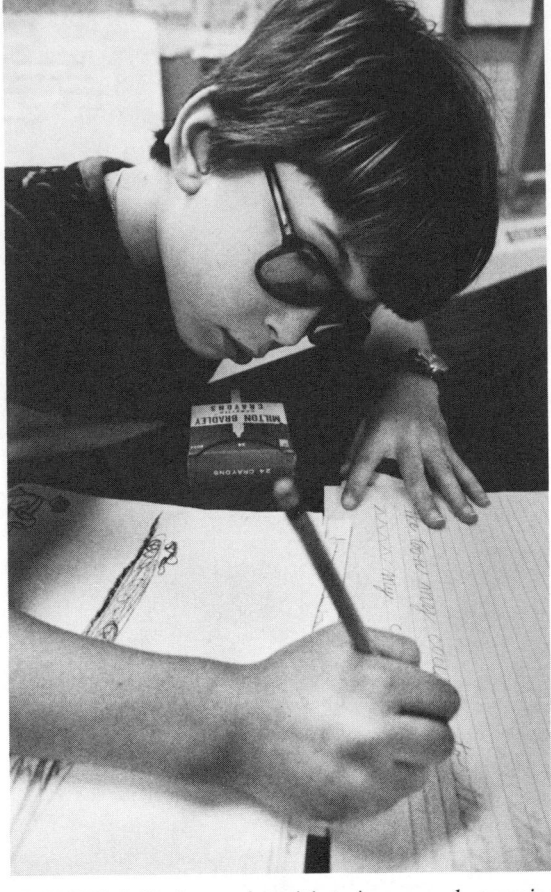

FIGURE 7.58 Journal writing is a good exercise for developing narrative awareness.

sonally significant, an event or a feeling for example. Often motivation for this task is provided by explaining that the journal is private and will not be corrected by the teacher, just shared.

The journals are often precise records of what students did from the time they left school to the time they went to bed. Included are the specifics of dinner and sometimes a recap of a television show that they watched. (*FIGURE 7.58*) It takes quite a bit of explanation and encouragement on the part of the teacher before a student effectively uses this written mode. Much of the difficulty stems from the student writer's inability to establish an initial intent, focus on it and select the critical material to discuss. He also may lack the linguistic structures needed for such expression. For example, instead of saying,

> "David got mad and threw Bill's books down the stairs. I suppose that Bill deserved it."

the student may give an extensive description of the situation, replete with dialogue which he hopes will convey his intent.

> "I saw David and Bill walking down the hall. Bill said, 'Nancy doesn't like you.' David said 'No. She likes me better.' Bill said, 'You are crazy.' David threw the books down the stairs. Bill is mean."

Reading other stories in journal entry form, or short novels with the same structure, helps to explain the task required.

One of the significant problems which surfaces in the reading and writing of journals and newspapers is that of narrative voice. To whom is one writing in a journal? Oneself? The teacher? No one? The question becomes most relevant when to *whom* one is writing determines *how* one writes. Part of this difficulty can be countered through programs with strong writing components. Writing activities which have a healthy balance in the lower grades of both public writing (charts, posters, etc.) and private writing (either dictation to teacher or writing to one specific reader) can lay a strong foundation for the issues which must be dealt with when beginning to recognize and respond to points of view in extended narrative discourse.

A specific activity helpful in breaking the pattern of recording direct discourse and relying on narratives chiefly composed of dialogue is to have one student read another student's journal entry and comment on it. The easiest task might be to have the reader paraphrase what he has read in a classmate's or other writer's journal.

After paraphrasing the student should be able to hold the journal entry in mind and comment on the writer's intent. For example, after reading "The Rime of the Ancient Mariner" by Samuel Coleridge the student might say, "I suppose that the Mariner is very sorry about killing the bird." Or, commenting on Manny's journal entry concerning his argument at basketball practice John concludes, "I suppose that Manny won't come to practice today. It appears that Manny was still upset when he wrote this last night." Numerous conversational activities can be used to draw the reader's attention to first listening to a speaker and then commenting on the speaker as well.

By specifying and limiting the topic of the journal entry itself, the teacher can focus greater attention on the narrative voice. For example, the student can create a snapshot journal in which he picks one thing he has seen during the day, freezes the moment in time and describes it. Again, the reader of the journal is required to speculate about the import of such an entry. Given that Nancy describes a lonely old woman picking up a heavy shopping bag, the reader can respond,

> "I believe that Nancy felt sorry for the lady," or
> "I suppose that Nancy wanted to help the old woman," or
> "It appears that this snapshot made Nancy feel bad."

Critical reading demands the very same uses of complex inferencing. Unless a student has had experience with creative writing and manipulation of style and focus, it is difficult for him to imagine something read as the product, expression or art of an author.

Students have read many types of material up until now; short stories, poems, biographies, fantasies, and perhaps they have even done thematic comparisons in writing. For instance, in the lower grades the students may read such works as Silverstein's The Giving Tree (1964) and Oscar Wilde's The Selfish Giant (1963), their themes being sharing or, globally, character's growing wiser. Perhaps in middle school they have studied the theme of death or loss by reading Charlotte's Webb, or e.e. cummings' "a leaf," or Paul Simon's "Old Friends." However, the interaction up until now has been an explicit one between the character, or dramatic action in the story or poem, and the reader. Readers now must develop more efficiency in reading through comprehension of increasingly complex, implicit information. Previously in reading, the students were asked to put themselves in the character's place with the question, "What would you have done?", or to anticipate the character's next decision, "What would you do?" This type of work can now be expanded by having the student pick another character in the story and retell the story through that character's eyes.

The actual preparation for this identification was begun in the earlier years through dramatization. When role playing or acting out a story, students become the characters they are asked to portray. A scene which lends itself nicely to such dramatization is from the story The Three Wishes (Craig, 1968) where the husband returns home with no food and the wife becomes very angry. Even though the young child knows the whole story and knows that the wife is punished for her stupidity and greed (a sausage grows from her nose), the student is usually enthusiastic about immersing himself in the wife's anger. This type of activity is common in the elementary grades as a way of adopting a person's perspective or point of view. However, carrying this over to written form is usually limited to reporting a dialogue.

In these earlier settings the dramatic action is foregrounded while interpretations of character and intent remain elementary. Readers who can pick a character from a story and retell a scene or the entire story from that character's perspective are singled out. The exercise is not purely one of writing gymnastics but also permits students to see the subtle process of character creation in their reading. In this stage of more complex understanding, journal writing takes on new functions and forms. The task becomes one of turning the snapshot journal into a type of empathy log.

Returning to the initial journal entry of the old woman picking up a heavy bag, the writer can either use the direct discourse approach and talk as though he or she were the old woman picking up the bag:

"I wish someone would help me carry this bag. It is so heavy. My fingers hurt. I can't walk very far."

or a classmate may hypothesize about the old woman:

"I suppose the woman is very tired. It must be so difficult for her in the cold weather."

Attending to how characters are conceived by the writer and apprehended by the reader is critical in the development of both reading and writing.

COMPLEX LITERARY FORMS

There is usually great emphasis on quantity of reading and especially writing in the school curriculum; the more words you can read or write, the better. The student therefore sees the reading or writing task quantitatively and is not motivated to use a more efficient system of organization; one which requires comprehension of linguistic structures, such as nominalization and deletions, as well as comprehension of text forms which make similar conceptual and cognitive demands. The book Come Again in the Spring (Kennedy, 1976) about an old man's successful escape from the figure of Death opens with ". . . . *A solitary figure trudging through the forest* . . ." rather than "*The solitary figure who was trudging through the forest* . . ." This structural deletion condenses the perception of events and character, creating a snapshot image easily held in the mind's eye.

Highly imagistic forms in text seem to be good vehicles for introducing fundamentals of imagery and perspective. For example, Haiku's compact structure makes it manageable and, at the same time, draws attention to the precise selectivity used by the writer. Students are challenged to take a snapshot of life and with words give that image meaning and import. It is a form which requires total concentration. Hearing-impaired students are often asked to produce extended narrative paragraphs and consequently find it difficult to encapsulate many thoughts into forms and structures which require a controlled selection and combination of words. By looking and feeling more closely, students can train their focus.

The wind blew many yellow
pages around—
Butterflies.

The sun died but
it will come back—
The life cycle.

My father looks into the oven
shock—
A mushroom is growing.

Imagery becomes a very strong tool for both writer and reader since information is no longer stated explicitly. In critical reading one perceives an overall controlling image in a passage, relying on the images within the story rather than the specific acts or content. Thus, reading and writing become more efficient. This use of imagery is important in apprehension of character in prose fiction.

Not only are characters described in the text, but characters' attributes and vehicles that carry them are also revealed. For instance, the reader first meets Milo of The Phantom Tollbooth (Juster, 1961) in a passage where he is explicity described by the omniscient narrator.

"*There was once a boy named Milo who didn't know what to do with himself–not just sometimes, but always. When he was in school he longed to be out, and when he was out he longed to be in. On the way he thought about coming home, and coming home he thought about going. Wherever he was he wished he were somewhere else, and when he got there he wondered why he'd bothered. Nothing really interested him – least of all the things that should have*" (p. 9).

The character Milo is explicitly described in this passage, as opposed to the character of Sam Gribly from My Side of the Mountain (George, 1959) who is shown implicitly.

"*My bed is on the right as you enter, and is made of ash slats and covered with deer skins. On the left is a small fireplace about knee high. It is of clay and stones. It has a chimney that leads the smoke out through a knothole..The air coming in is bitter cold. It must be below zero outside, and yet I can sit here inside my tree and write with bare hands"* (p. 316).

As Parker (1969) points out, *"these details of Sam's environment on the wintry mountainside reveal Sam's resourcefulness in the world of nature"* (p. 23).

Along with adolescent literature with its very present first person narration, students are increasingly required to comprehend textbook material that demonstrates a very different style of writing. It is often claimed that this type of reading material is dry because of its preoccupation with information and lack of narrative voice. However, one function of textbook language is the achievement of objectivity and a preciseness of focus.

For instance, a typical social studies text dealing with Admiral Richard E. Byrd might read, *"Exploration of the continent and scientific analysis of data obtained there were the projects of the 1957–58 'operation deep freeze'."* The focus is not on Byrd but on what he did. The actor, Byrd, is deleted as the nominalized action becomes the focus of reader attention.

Or, from a textbook on the Age of the Renaissance (Shapiro, 1961), a description of this era appears as, *"It was as if the dead were being awakened. . . The living were awakening too, awakening from a long sleep and dark dreams of the Middle Ages. So great was the awakening that it seemed as if all mankind was being reborn"* (p. 8). While in the first two sentences people are awakening, the focus of the third sentence shifts from the acts of people to a description of the act itself (the awakening - a nominalization).

The nominalized form can also function to change new information into old thereby shifting the focus. The concluding statement in the book Arrow to the Sun (McDermott, 1977) is: *"The people celebrated his return in the Dance of Life."* Stylistically, to rewrite this would create; "He returned to the people and they celebrated," or "The people celebrated because he returned to earth."

In an attempt to simplify one most commonly rewrites and restructures by subjectifying the text or placing the agent of the action back into the scene. Thus, one explains that Macbeth and Lady Macbeth were ambitious and dissatisfied and discusses what they did because they were ambitious. But how does one move away from their acts to discuss their condition and to generalize about ambition? This demands some functional use of abstract superordinate categories that encompass such concepts as ambition or loneliness.

The Tinman's kindness, the Lion's courage, and the Strawman's loyality are the targets of reward in The Wizard of Oz. Without that focus, it becomes difficult to universalize and recognize these traits in others. The traits become, of necessity, abstract concepts or symbols (a lion as a symbol for courage) for the reader so they may be specified somewhere else along the way, in another story or in one's own experiences.

This type of objectifying can also prevent the reader's stigmatizing or misjudging persons based on one act. For example, a fair coach who shows anger and frustration is often labeled by the adolescent as "an angry person." The fair coach thus becomes unfair, for the student is unable to speak about the action without subjectifying it. The reader must learn to separate and analyze a person apart from his act; to weigh each by its own import. For adolescents this separation of person from act is a significant problem.

The functions of objectifying will eventually expand the reader's ability to generalize a common attribute as uniquely manifested, for instance, in three different characters. Thus, the quality of ambition in "The Three Little Pigs," "Icarus and Daedalus," and "Macbeth" is linked despite the diversity of their actions: Daedalus flies to the Gods, the Pigs run away from home, and Macbeth kills a king, yet the ambition of each can be abstracted.

This chapter has tried to show how comprehension of more complex linguistic and literary structures contributes to the meaningfulness of the reading and writing experience. Mastery in the use of these more complex organizational systems continues the development of a generative process with which the student may approach new information with confidence and commitment.

SUGGESTED READINGS

READING AND LITERATURE

Frye, N. *An anatomy of criticism: Four essays.* Princeton: Princeton University Press, 1957.
Kohlberg, L. The child as moral philosopher. *Psychology Today,* September, 1968.
Tucker, N. How children respond to fiction. *Children's Literature in Education,* November, 1972.

LINGUISTICS

Chafe, W. *Meaning and the structure of language.* Chicago: University of Chicago Press, 1970.
Green, G.M. *Semantics and syntactic regularity.* Bloomington, IL: Indiana University Press, 1974.

ACKNOWLEDGMENTS

QUOTES

Page 113 From unit prepared by Susan Kondas and Christina Montecalvo, Rhode Island School for the Deaf.

Page 118 From "Dreams" by Langston Hughes. Copyright © 1932 by Alfred A. Knopf, Inc., and renewed copyright © by Langston Hughes. Reprinted from *The Dream Keeper and Other Poems* by Langston Hughes with permission by Alfred A. Knopf, Inc.

Page 118 From *The Panther and the Lash: Poems of Our Times* by Langston Hughes. Copyright © 1951 by Langston Hughes, Reprinted with permission by Alfred A. Knopf, Inc.

Chapter 8

The Secondary School Experience

Development Versus Remediation

The hearing-impaired high school student may be the most language aware of any student. He is aware of what he can read, cannot read, and what he has to read; what he cannot say clearly and in what situations. He is also aware that teachers are aware of the limitations in his language abilities.

Our greatest sense of urgency comes when the student enters high school defeatedly proclaiming "me lousy language." To the teacher it is a request interpreted as: "Teacher, you've got it all up there. Now, you've got a semester or two or three; can't you just take the time and give it all to me?"

The pattern of instruction commonly followed by teachers can be described as follows: the teacher assumes the burden of teaching the student all the language and concepts that he does not have and, when the language work isn't paying off, tries to feed him the concepts in spite of the language. When progress is predictably slow there is then the urge to turn to survival skills. Fulfilling such an urge is too often to turn toward remediation and away from development.

This sense of urgency is most acute in the secondary program. Teachers faced with the final responsibility of preparing students for what is to come after graduation perceive their role as educators in significantly different ways from those of lower or middle school teachers. All secondary school teachers are conscious of and take some active responsibility for the young person's future beyond the school experience. Perhaps it is unfair but somehow the secondary school teacher is not only held accountable for his or her own class at the time of instruction, but also for what happens to the student after graduation.

Because the teacher has the student for three, possibly four more years, there is a sense of urgency that, regardless of what happened before, it all has to come together now. Language has to be straightened out and work habits and study skills have to be developed. If there has been little emphasis on speech, then oral communication must improve so the student is prepared for the outside world. In addition there are the volumes of information and skills the student should have before leaving school. And, compounding all that makes up the secondary school experience, there is the nature of adolescence.

Added to these difficult considerations is the ever-present dilemma of finding appropriate language and reading materials for these students, for so much of the subject content area depends on comprehension of information obtained through books. In fact the language problems of secondary school hearing-impaired students present teachers of all subject areas with unique problems in teaching and curriculum design. The actual functioning of the classroom depends upon efficient functioning in language and this problem exists independent of subject area. Yet, when involved in a teaching workshop on language, the vocational teacher is often heard to say, "This really doesn't concern me, I teach woodworking." Then, as the discussion of language proceeds, that same teacher may observe, "You know, my students have great problems following directions. The directions say 'plane a face side' or 'cut the wood to the required length.' The students read it but don't do it." And yet the students usually know what the task involves, and once the directions are explained they immediately proceed to do a fine job.

The issue is not one of skill with machinery but skill with the language that is required. Following directions requires comprehension of imperative structures and, as pointed out earlier, students often are unaware of the essential difference between declarative, interrogative and imperative sentences. The imperative structures are unavoidable in the day-to-day functioning of the vocational, math and science classrooms and, because of this language gap, teaching can be not only inefficient but impossible. Under these circumstances the teacher, by having to explain the task, defeats a major goal of creating more independent learners. Thus, teaching language is the responsibility of all members of the secondary staff and not the sole responsibility of the English teacher.

Another problem unique to the secondary level is the student who has a systematic grammar, perhaps a complex one, but still has gaps in terms of morphological accuracy or specific syntactic processes (e.g., topicalization for semantic focus). There is often the temptation to correct or remediate what is wrong, independent of other developmental processes. Again this problem is often left for the English teacher to solve, but as one vocational teacher at the Rhode Island School for the Deaf has noted, teaching the difference between *machine* as a verb and *machine* as a noun is his business too. For the art teacher dealing with morphological changes such as *cube/cubism,* there is no time to wait for the English teacher to find a spot for *-ism* in the curriculum. At the secondary level, higher level gaps in a student's language mastery are still gaps that affect all academic areas.

A third problem unique to the secondary level programs for the hearing impaired are the late beginners; those students who come from improper placements and have gone unnoticed for years, or more recently, immigrant students who have had little or no education in their homeland. It is this problem as well as the others noted that brings up a very basic question about work at the secondary level: is the teacher's responsibility one of continuing (or recapitulating) development, or is the task one of remediation? The dichotomy between development and remediation may be too narrow, for the teacher's task surely involves aspects of both. Though it cannot be denied that there are language problems evident at this level that reflect gaps and weaknesses requiring remediation, the upper school language program should still remain an integral aspect of the developmental process of language acquisition. While there remains the task of diagnosing the needs of advanced students, the danger lies in designing a curriculum with only remediation in mind. Such programs assume that the information has been taught correctly at some previous time in the student's school experience and that the student has failed to learn.

Herbert Kohl's (1973) statement in regard to reading remediation is true of remediation in general:

"The assumption that a student needs remedial help if he or she has not learned to read needs to be examined. First of all, if someone has not acquired a skill there is nothing to remediate. . . . If a person who has not learned to read can be considered as someone to be taught or helped for the first time, then the whole problem of guilt or failure disappears and with it the need for a special place to deal with failure" (p. 14).

The following sections were written by secondary school teachers at the Rhode Island School for the Deaf. They illustrate attempts to deal with the urgency and frustration of the later years of a student's schooling by maintaining a developmental and creative approach to teaching.

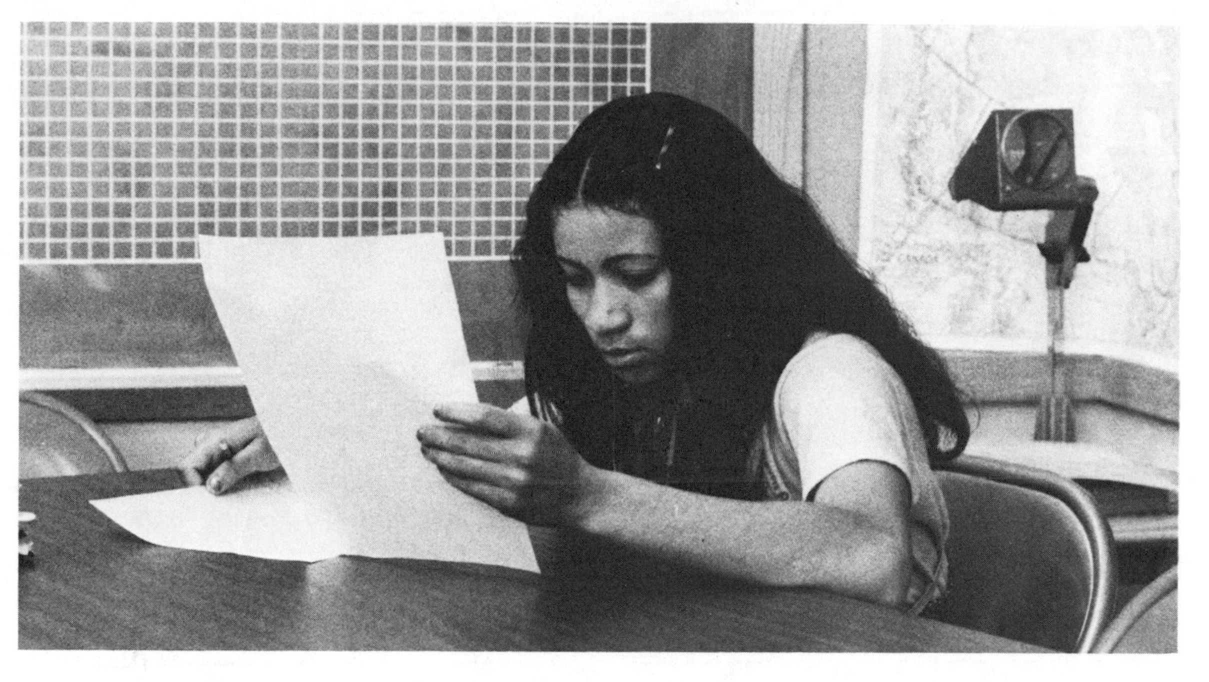

Curriculum Planning for the Late Beginner

One of the most perplexing questions asked by teachers on the secondary level is what to do about the late beginner – the transfers from other programs, adolescents coming to this country for the first time, the young person who has never had any schooling. The solution to these unfortunate circumstances is usually heavy doses of remedial training focusing upon the young person's deficits rather than upon his strengths.

The developmental approach, however, can still apply. It is a matter of assessing what cognitive and linguistic abilities the late starter might have and then using these abilities as a starting point. The aim is to fill in past gaps by creating possibilities for growth.

One of the diagnostic tasks of the secondary school teacher is to find out whether the late beginner has established a system of linguistic representation at all, however primitive or inefficient. If the student has acquired a grammar which is, in fact, productive (generative), there is then much for a teacher to build on. However, if there is no apparent sense for syntax but rather a randomly connected string of vocabulary, it seems little can be done until a basic grammar is established. This does not mean that the content work has to be simple or elementary, but that the sentences used to carry the content are initially structured to also convey the linguistic patterns necessary for the establishment of syntactic structure. We see this need most often among 10- or 11-year-old students from other countries. If they have had any schooling, they usually have a small set of vocabulary in their home language but no sense of syntax.

One very successful experience with a group of late beginning students is summarized by a teacher who was not only able to accomplish meaningful content and conceptual goals but also helped his students move into a generative language system.

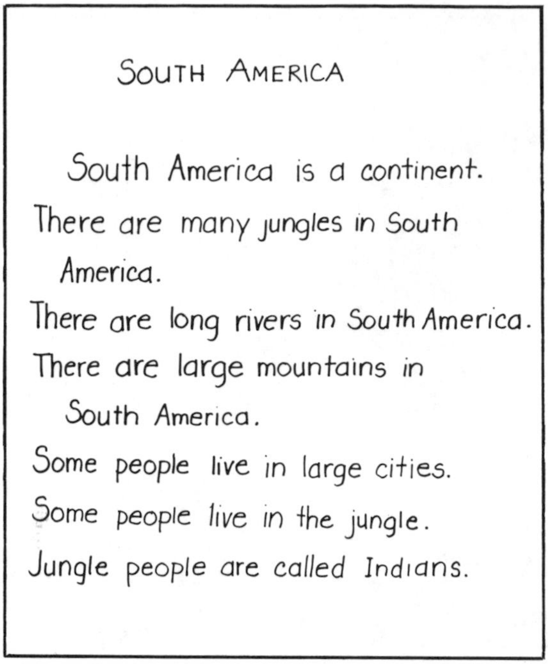

SOUTH AMERICA

South America is a continent.
There are many jungles in South America.
There are long rivers in South America.
There are large mountains in South America.
Some people live in large cities.
Some people live in the jungle.
Jungle people are called Indians.

FIGURE 8.59 The unit was introduced with a chart dealing with some of the general geographical and demographical characteristics of the South American continent.

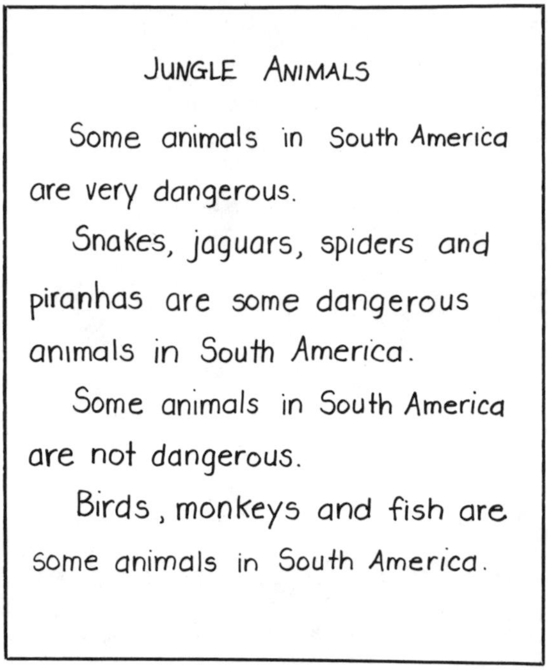

JUNGLE ANIMALS

Some animals in South America are very dangerous.
Snakes, jaguars, spiders and piranhas are some dangerous animals in South America.
Some animals in South America are not dangerous.
Birds, monkeys and fish are some animals in South America.

We moved to a more specific discussion of jungles, their topography, rainfall and temperature. Students prepared color-coded graphs to represent this information.

by Charles Girard

In 1973 I was confronted with providing a social studies program for an adolescent group of hearing-impaired immigrant students. These children had little or no past experience with school, let alone English! Also, their native language experience was limited.

The initial problem besides communication was finding materials that would motivate a young teenager to work on developing language, reading and speech skills. Once appropriate materials were located, the goal was to provide the students with the necessary skills to recognize the syntax or word order of kernel sentences. Upon mastery, the students were to combine these kernels to form complex sentences and by the following year to produce simple paragraphs.

To accomplish this I needed a high-interest, almost exotic educational vehicle. I selected the Kaingang Indians of South America and the aborigines of the Australian outback. Though separated by 10,000 miles, both groups are dependent upon their environment for survival and face the problem of an encroaching alien civilization. Because my own students were strangers in an alien culture they related personally to the materials. (*FIGURE 8.59*)

The materials were presented in carefully prepared steps that used language charts as the primary diagnostic and educational tool, supplemented by films and manipulative activities such as map and graph making. The class time was divided into 30 minutes for language arts and speech and 20 minutes for project activities.

Was it successful? The students are now three years older and juniors in our high school. They are involved in my World History class that prepares them for the integrated senior art and literature program.

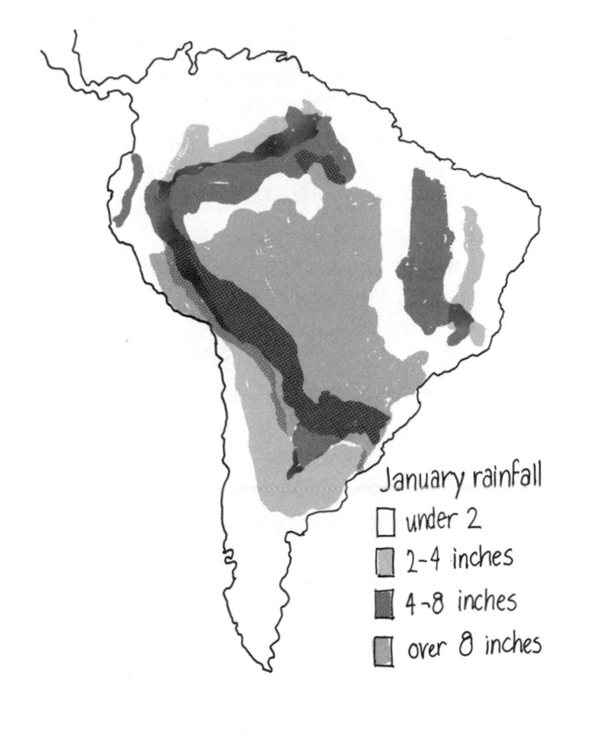

JUNGLES

Jungles are very hot.

Jungles are very wet.

Many different animals live
in the jungle.

There are great rivers in the jungle.

Trees grow very quickly. The
jungle is very dense.

A third chart on exotic jungle animals led to an involved study of the Kaingang Indians.

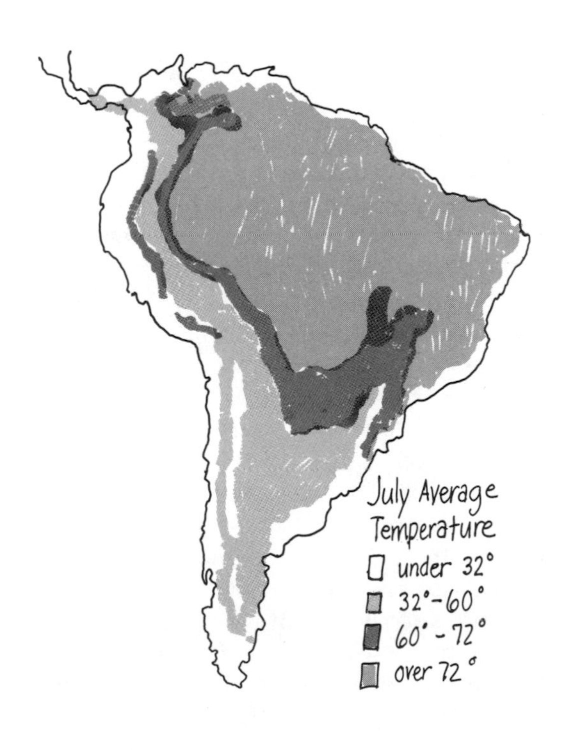

The Process of Interdisciplinary Planning

The preceding description was one that dealt with the late beginner. The following selection speaks to a different issue; interdisciplinary planning on the secondary level.

One way to help students and teachers understand that language does not belong only in the English classroom but is a part of all areas of learning is to have one or two teachers in different subject areas explore together the interrelationship of language to find the most effective methods of instruction. In the following section, English and math teachers discuss and evaluate their efforts to use diagnostic teaching activities to delineate specific areas of language and cognitive development. They also describe their approach to issues of development and remediation. This type of effort reflects a commitment to teaching through language rather than in spite of language.

by Jeffrey Cole and Judith Gilman Garland

In Chapter 5 it was noted that "*. . . . the language of elementary mathematics word problems is exceedingly complex. . . and while students often have the computational skills called for by the problem, they may not have the receptive syntactic ability to understand the linguistic expression of the problem.*" It may also be true that they do not have the necessary cognitive schemas to analyze and comprehend the semantic structure of the problem.

This type of difficulty is especially true at the high school level. Here they are not only confronted with difficult mathematical word problems in the shop areas and algebra courses but are faced with comprehending, analyzing, evaluating and generalizing complex concepts and large quantities of data in other subject areas as well. Without the concomitant cognitive strategies and schemas, the linguistic input for handling the data and concepts is generally an exercise in rote memorization. To address these cognitive deficits and the resulting faculty frustrations, a different high school program was initiated.

The still-evolving program is being taught simultaneously in English (literature) and in math to the freshman class. The original rationale for the program was to keep the two freshman classes intact for a number of periods (English, math, social studies and science) so that a common cognitive and conceptual content could be generalized across subject areas. It was felt that such a procedure would break down the subject-teacher content confinement; allow for enhanced reinforcement, expansion and generalization of conceptual content; and, most importantly, allow for development of broad cognitive strategies and schemas.

The content area was based on a four-year high school curriculum which focused on the themes of identity, conflict, change and commitment. Although these are not mutually exclusive themes, identity was chosen as the first year focal point. A rapid listing of the components of a sense of identity soon yielded more than a semester's worth of material. To winnow out the significant factors and help each of us direct our classroom teaching, each idea was expanded into a full sentence describing what the student should know by the end of the semester. (*FIGURE 8.60*) This expansion also helped to clarify our perceptions of each item. We specified what was meant by each concept, arrived at a common understanding of each, and determined what would be useful concepts for the

INITIAL IDENTITY OUTLINE

I. IDENTITY
   A. Autonomy
      1. Uniqueness
      2. Decision making
         a) responsibility for decision
         b) risk taking
         c) rationalization
         d) validity of information
   B. Trust
      1. Relationship
         a) respect
         b) responsibility to other person
         c) sharing—interpersonal tension—risk
      2. Suspended disbelief
      3. Acceptance vs. doubt
      4. Decision making—objective vs. subjective
   C. Accomplishment
      1. Success
      2. Sense of worth
      3. Productivity
      4. Perception of role
         a) defenses
            1. conscious vs. unconscious; truth vs. deception
            2. defense mechanisms
         b) functionality
            1. perspective; point of view

FIGURE 8.60 Initial identity outline

students to develop. For example, decision making became *one's unique ability to make decisions to enable one to become autonomous.* This was then further broken down into subordinate and superordinate conceptual sentences. Any concept that could not be expanded into a commonly acceptable sentence or which did not seem to have real utility for the student was shelved as not being of immediate relevance. The sentences that remained were then put into a logical developmental outline to be used simultaneously by all of the teachers involved. (*FIGURE 8.61*)

CONCEPTUAL STATEMENTS
Expanded From Initial Identity Outline

I. IDENTITY: A sense and acceptance of self, which is a changing product of one's growth in a culture and environment and which influences that culture and environment.
   A. Autonomy: An awareness of one's uniqueness which enables one to become self-sufficient.
      1. Uniqueness: One's integration of common events during a life cycle produces individual differences.
      2. Decision making: One's unique ability to make decisions enables one to become autonomous.
         a) Decision making involves choice which involves risk because one doesn't always:
            1. know the consequences.
            2. have sufficient and valid information to make comfortable decisions.
         b) One's ability to know the consequences and have enough information is influenced by:
            1. one's background.
            2. one's opinion.
         c) Conformity and defense mechanisms (rationalization, sublimation and displacement) serve to lessen the impact of the consequences. Having made a decision, one is therefore responsible for accepting the consequences.

FIGURE 8.61 Examples of conceptual statements expanded from initial identity outline

After evaluating the incoming students' experiences and abilities it was decided that the first concept to be introduced would be decision making. This was not presented with the "values determine decisions" orientation but from the point of view of choice and possible consequences or risks. In specifying these concepts, a common language base evolved which could be used in each subject area. Cognitively we began with the analysis and evaluation of the decision process and strategies for classification.

In the classrooms the initial focus was on the students' abilities to respond to questions. Given any question the students had to determine the type of question asked, choose an appropriate response type and the appropriate information specific to that question. Specific subject area examples were easy to find as every question asked involving either plot, geography, history, vertebrate anatomy, or building a cabinet required a student to make some sort of decision regarding an appropriate answer. For example, analysis of the decision process in math involved having the students listen to or read a question concerning the shapes and patterns that form tesselations or tiling patterns (for example, "Do octagons form tiling patterns?"). They then had to decide what was an appropriate response (initially "yes" or "no"), determine the consequences of each decision, weigh the risks and form a conclusion.

In English the process was applied to literature skills. The following focal points were considered as vehicles through which decision making would be developed.

(1) Point of view and author's voice
(2) Stylistic variations
(3) Characterization

As we were attempting the program with a freshman class which had never taken an intensive literature course, possibilities (1) and (2) were temporarily ruled out as too involved and sophisticated and too dependent on highly developed language skills. It was determined that the literature classes would start off with a study of characterization.

A vocabulary list was compiled for discussion of the literary aspects of characterization and the short stories and poems presented were built around obvious character decisions, such as the short story, "Through the Tunnel" by Doris Lessing and the poem, "The Road Not Taken" by Robert Frost. In some of the stories the consequences of the decisions made by the characters were more blatant than others, but the variety and the subtlety in the poetry, for example, was essential to reinforce generalization of this kind of observation and understanding.

Through discussions of each phase of the program's initial section, we discovered many linguistic structures that the students needed to know to fully appreciate the cognitive focus of the classes. For example, the first structured language form presented in the English class came out of the empirical/nonempirical data discussions of the math class. It was essential for the students' progress to demonstrate and develop language categories exemplified by the empirical "I know" versus the nonempirical "I believe" and their negative counterparts, "I don't know" and "I don't think so." By contrasting the different language forms, this particular language lesson was taught along with the development of characterization in literature.

At this point another decision-making process was introduced that paralleled the "I'm not sure" or "I don't know" language structures. When students encountered insufficient information or an uncomfortable risk level, the procedure became one of formulating and testing a hypothesis before a decision was made and the students committed themselves to a response. If the test disproved the hypothesis or the risk was too great, a feedback loop was to be initiated consisting of a period of study or information gathering and the formulation of a new hypothesis. Once the hypothesis was felt to be adequate and the resulting risks within acceptable limits, a decision was made, a response given and the consequences awaited. Faced with any question, the student now had a choice of processes and was continually faced with the decision of which one to use.

It was at this point that we began getting away from the original identity outline and focusing more and more on the cognitive skills and schemas. As the amount of work-

SET THEORY AND CROSS SUBJECT COGNITIVE SKILLS

ELEMENTS OF SET THEORY—Cognitive Skills or Concepts Addressed Within the Unit.

set—*classifying* diverse elements on the basis of common attributes

criteria—*abstracting* out a set of common attributes which are present in every instance

counterexample—exceptions used to test the *validity and sufficiency* of the set criteria and to *evaluate* an *overgeneralization*

forms of notation—choosing an appropriate *form of representation* from those available

roster notation—objective listing of the instances or *examples*

description notation—forming a *generalization* which precisely states the set criteria and therefore *defines* the set

set builder notation—*analysis* of each instance with respect to the set criteria

Venn diagrams—visual-spatial analogs for specifying and examining set *relationships*

Universal set—*superordinate classification* from which one possible set is chosen

null set/nonempty set, finite set/infinite set—*comparison* and *classification* of contrastive pairs

subset, proper subset, improper subset, equal sets, disjoint sets—*reasoning* through *analysis* and *evaluation* of set relationships

complement—*negative classification* where an instance is not a member of a given set

union and intersection of sets—*divergent and convergent concept relationships*

FIGURE 8.62 Set theory and cross subject cognitive skills

ing data within each subject area increased, the students began to encounter the normal dilemma of not being able to remember every instance of a concept or theme. They also had difficulty in understanding what constituted sufficient information and in formulating hypotheses. Thus, we began looking for describable and valid patterns within the data and then formulating the resultant criteria into abstract and generalizable statements. The classroom question then changed from "Can you make a decision . . .?" to "Can you make a generalization about this data?"

However, it became apparent from the students' responses that there were some deficits in their ability to generalize. We had taught "generalization" and, though the students were beginning to generalize within a class, they were not transferring the skill from class to class. This was partly a linguistic problem in that the students were still wrestling with the form of a general statement, but mainly it was a cognitive problem; one that was not immediately remediable if the students had not fully entered into the formal operational stage of cognition. We had no choice but to be patient and continue building and reinforcing, waiting for the students to integrate their language competence and performance. So, with another turn of the spiral we returned to decision making.

Decisions involving empirical data often include classification processes. Comparing similar attributes helps to organize bits of data into meaningful groups. In order to recognize patterns or generate generalizable statements, one must be able to analyze the data in terms of previously acquired sets of knowledge. This is as true for plot comparisons in literature and cross-cultural comparisons in social studies as it is for data generated in science or math. To address these skills we began a cross-subject study of set theory. The bulk of the teaching was, of course, relegated to math but each skill and concept was used and practiced in the other subject areas. (*FIGURE 8.62*)

The emphasis was on the use of "set criteria" to classify data and to introduce the logical relationships between the sets of data. The students had to learn that these criteria must be precise enough to include only the logically inclusive instances and exclude all others. For example, given the set (soccer, basketball, track, field hockey) the description *sports* could also include polo, whereas *sports played at the Rhode Island School for the Deaf* could not. One process for analyzing set criteria employs the use of counter-examples. In the above example *polo* serves to further define the set criteria. The students now would have to refine their linguistic skills to state general criteria and to evaluate and perhaps challenge stated criteria.

To address the problem of examples (instances) being synonymous with definitions (set criteria), different ways of representing sets were introduced. Sets can be described, among other ways, in terms of their criteria (description notation) or by listing all of the members (roster notation). As new data were compared with existing sets, the students began to combine cognitive skills with their linguistic abilities. The students then classified the new instances by comparing their attributes with the set criteria and we began to expect supportive reasoning for the decisions made.

As the work in the math class began focusing on the use of criteria for making classification decisions, the English class moved to exposure of the symbolic meaning of poetry. "Support your answer" became the rule and the constant question in both English and math classes became "Why?" Each day carried a double opportunity for understanding and practicing the same skill of supportive reasoning. As the students were required to compare several stories and poems, they began to develop generalizations about the characters, the author's advice (voice), the specific symbols of poetry and the overall symbolic meaning.

The students did not produce these generalizations spontaneously. Though given contrived exposure, the generalizations were not evident to the students until directly elicited by the teacher. The skill of thinking in terms of generalization needed to be developed to the point where we taught the word *generalization* itself and described how they had been doing it. Later, as the students gained competence, questioning alone became a sufficient instigator. The advantages of having abundant examples in several subject areas where the material is naturally diverse were enormous.

To further the students' skill in abstracting generalizable criteria from data we began to focus attention on the relationships between things. In math we began a series of lessons on relations including such things as the diagraming of family relations and the mapping of functions and Cartesian products; in science we graphed an experiment on angular acceleration; in English we discussed the relationships between different symbols and the expression of each in their respective stories. As additional reinforcement of the concept of relationship, we used examples from each others' classes. Contrary to the expectations that this would result in massive confusion for the students, it seemed to make it easier for them. The material almost became irrelevant as they focused on using the concept.

Throughout this process we found it both necessary and extremely beneficial to engage in an almost constant dialogue. We discussed our progress toward our goals; the vocabulary, examples and materials that we used; and the students' successes and difficulties with the materials. One such dialogue produced the observation that, whereas the students were indeed using supportive reasoning, their reasoning was not always valid. Further discussions of this frustrating observation led to an introductory unit on logical thinking and persuasion.

During the first few classes on logical persuasion, the students used stereotyped generalizations as points of argument. For example, in an exercise on persuading a male classmate to cut his hair the argument was given that "girls don't like long hair." Many such generalizations would have proven false if tested as hypotheses and, although we were excited to see the students using generalizations, we questioned their understanding of the power of the language of generalization for organizing and viewing the world (for example, stereotypes). In relating our concern to the secondary science teacher we made a timely discovery. The students' assignment in science was a reading exercise to test their understanding and production of the language style used to express a hypothesis, a skill that had been introduced and partially developed last year.

Ensuring that the aspects of the lessons essential to their science learning would be covered, the English classes set about to develop the students' awareness of the categories of language styles that were in conflict in their production of hypotheses.

It was not long before the students were able to identify a hypothesis as different from a specific statement; the area of difficulty now lay in the students' production. As it was now quite obvious to the students that the two teachers were concentrating on the same issue, it became advantageous to readopt the role of English teacher and point out the style of the language that hypothesizing requires. By focusing attention on this specific linguistic awareness, the students were able to see the task of hypothesis production as twofold: that it must contain the relationship being considered and it must also be stated in a specific manner. Soon after this lesson the students were identifying hypotheses in other classes without being asked to do so. Application of their new knowledge in various disciplines encouraged us to believe that true generalization was indeed taking place.

Simultaneously in math the lessons were focusing on simple and compound statements and truth tables. Here the students

STATEMENTS AND VENN DIAGRAMS

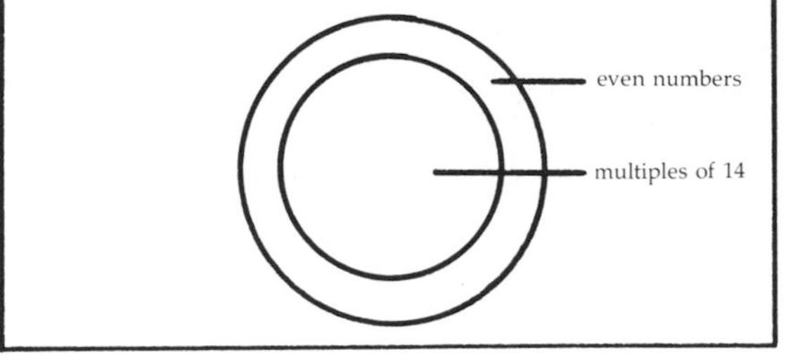

Statement:
Multiples of 14 are even numbers.

Set Language:
The set of numbers which are multiples of 14 is a subset of the set of even numbers.

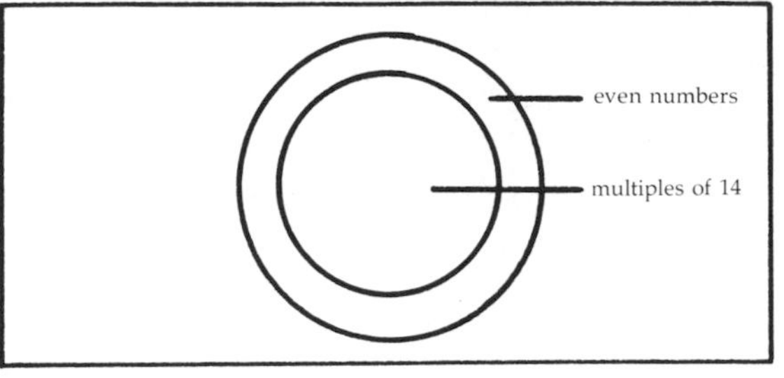

Statement:
X is an even number and it is less than 10. (X is a member of the set of natural numbers.)

Set Language:
In every instance X is a member of the intersection of the set of even numbers and the set of numbers less than 10.

FIGURE 8.63 Examples of statements and Venn diagrams

QUANTIFIERS AND THEIR VISUAL-SPATIAL REPRESENTATIONS

STATEMENT	SET LANGUAGE	DIAGRAM
Men are animals.	The set of all men is a subset of the set of animals.	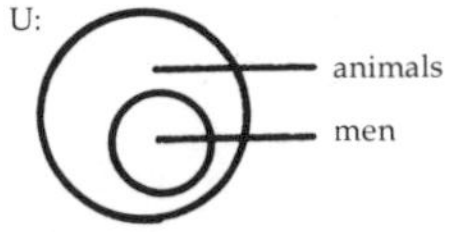 U: animals; men
Some students have cars.	The set of students intersects with the set of people who have cars.	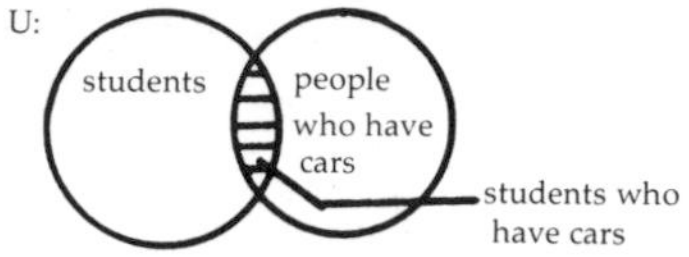 U: students; people who have cars; students who have cars
Many students play basketball.	The set of students intersects with the set of basketball players.	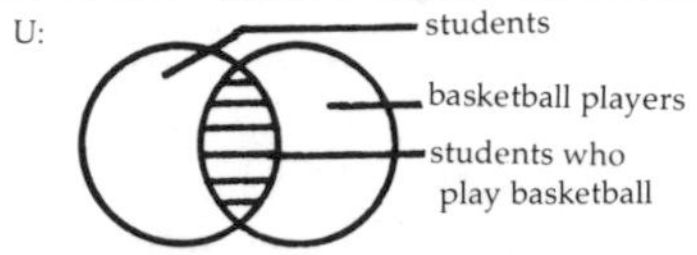 U: students; basketball players; students who play basketball
None of the odd numbers are even.	No member of the set of odd numbers is also a member of the set of even numbers.	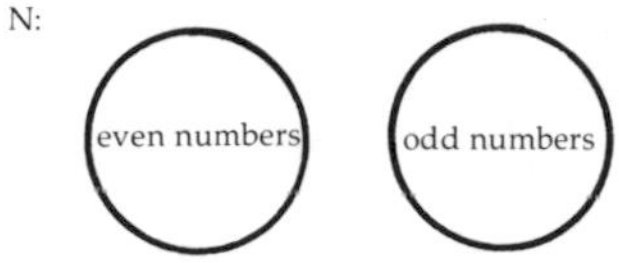 N: even numbers; odd numbers

FIGURE 8.64 Examples of statements using quantifiers and their visual-spatial representations

had to utilize their linguistic knowledge to analyze statements and specify the semantic relations with Venn diagrams. (*FIGURE 8.63*) To further their linguistic abilities the math class also became an English class with both conducting a series of lessons on quantifiers (all, some, no, none, . . .). Again, contrast played an important role in developing these concepts. (*FIGURE 8.64*)

At this point we were dealing with a number of concepts from different areas and the students were having difficulty in focusing on the critical math concepts of logical truth tables. Both the students and the math teacher became frustrated by the confusion and found it necessary to call a truce and begin the logic unit again. This time the students had had some exposure to the concepts being analyzed and we were able to draw on their abilities to formulate hypotheses and generalizations and to give supportive reasoning. To simplify the concepts and to eliminate the students' preconceptions of some of the linguistic and informational relationships in a given statement, a nonsense word statement was used. Now the students had to focus on the semantic/cognitive relationships specified by the statement and especially on the function of the quantifier. (*FIGURE 8.65*) This served both as an efficient and productive teaching technique and to reinforce and test their abilities to generalize.

At the beginning we had attempted to state our goals for the first semester. We are now a few weeks beyond the midterm and have not progressed on the identity theme. Given the change in the cognitive abilities of the students this does not seem of too great a concern. The program has been, and is, an ongoing process for both the students and the faculty. Its origins in the identity unit are not of vast significance. Nearly any program, unit or set of materials can be chosen as a start. Then once started, goals in cognition

Nonsense Word Statements Used to Emphasize Semantic-Cognitive Relationships

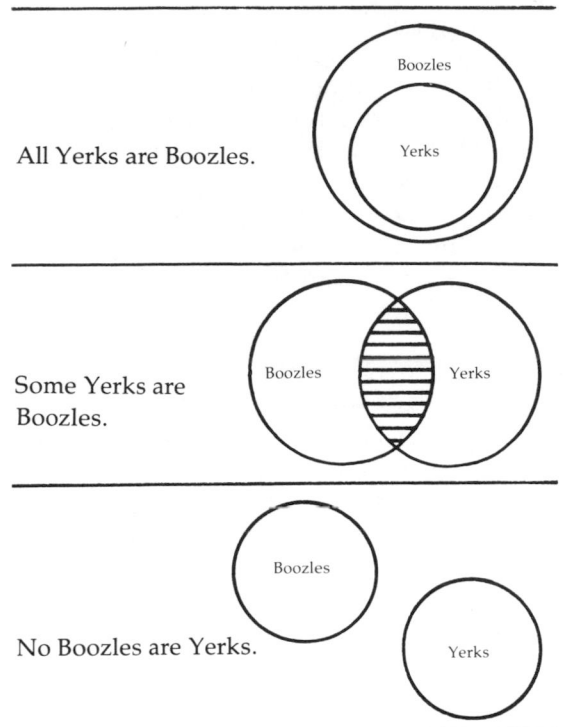

FIGURE 8.65 Nonsense word statements used to emphasize semantic-cognitive relationships

and thinking processes that meet the immediate needs of the students can be spiraled through it. There is no order as such, but as the program progresses the students will define what cognitive processes are needed and what specific language must be possessed to move ahead. However, going sideways to ensure a broader base upon which to build further cognitive and linguistic ability is not a negative or stationary step but an essential one. As a teacher this can be difficult and at times frustrating, but at the high school level, patience is necessary. (*FIGURE 8.66*)

We are dealing here with an attempt to cover, in a short span of time, what should take years to slowly develop. Students may

FIGURE 8.66

not reach the performance level for many months, or another teacher in a later year may see the results. The worth of such a program, however, does not need stating.

The program will be applied next year to a junior high class from the middle school. Eventually it will work its way down through the classes to where the children are at the concrete operational level. Obviously the materials used, the depth of coverage of any given concept and the method of presentation will be determined by the unique chemistry of a particular class and teacher. Indeed, even the youngest children who are functioning concretely can be exposed to and prepared for a future in-depth study of these concepts by utilizing appropriate enactive and iconic activities and materials.

Spiraling these concepts throughout the student's school life experience, with appropriate teacher manipulation of classroom situations and the timely exchange of examples and assignments (even classes and subjects), would help to ensure success and concept utility. With such flexibility and manipulation within an interdisciplinary process, and with skills enabling them to become more cognitively and linguistically competent individuals, the students should develop a growing sensitivity to learning.

Abstract Language and Literary Form

A constant frustration of the secondary school teacher is the literalness with which hearing-impaired students approach new information. Either something is literal or it is absurd and thus usually regarded as insignificant. Discussions of abstraction are difficult and what often occurs is that the teacher's abstractions or generalizations are perceived in a very concrete and specific way by the students. The literal one-to-one correspondences which have formed the student's learning patterns are most seriously reflected in their inability to perceive language as anything more than a concrete code of which they have only a tenuous understanding.

by Christina Zarcadoolas

As a new teacher I attempted to introduce singer-poet Paul Simon's work into the classroom. On initial reading the students saw "I Am a Rock" as nothing more than a geological exposé and "Bridge Over Troubled Water" simply as the personification of a bridge speaking to a commuter. We should expect this type of interpretation from younger children but it was a shock to hear it from young adults. The students' inability to understand the implied symbolism in the writings of Paul Simon indicated that work needed to be done on figurative language.

Symbolic language has many levels. It is one thing to say that "the tree was bent over like a dancer," and quite another to say that "the music of the wilderness rolled over the slight bulge of its belly." In a simile one is limited to comparing a tree to a dancer, but in the other (a metaphor) there is a reference to a wilderness that can make music; music that has locomotion and a tree which is much like a body - alive, vibrant and responsive. Unlike simile, metaphorical language gives us a sense of the willfulness of words as well as a sense of surprise and wonder as we see our world (and words) in varied new relationships.

We began by writing our own similes, comparing class members and inanimate objects. After weeks of discussion students could say that clouds are like horses galloping in the sky, or that eyes shine like rainbows. But simile confines the user to only two things held in tension. Both from reading the students' journals and holding in-class discussion I decided it was time to move from Haiku to some lyric poetry and metaphorical structures.

There was very little noticeable use of description through figurative language or evidence that the students were taking any creative risks with language. Their journals were simple accounts of their day-to-day activities; going to school, practicing sports, watching T.V. I was troubled by this lack of imagination and use of description. All things were recorded in the journal in the same way, with an occasional intrusion to tell what was seen or felt ("I won the race. I was very glad."). There was no showing of what was felt through use of description other than simple contrived simile constructions. It was clear that upon advancing from basal readers to reading literature the students hadn't changed their way of reading or their goals for reading or for writing. They had simply adopted a strategy for discarding descriptive language structures and comparisons in very much the same way they would discard a difficult, unfamiliar vocabulary word.

The move to lyric poetry was an attempt to bring more immediacy to the issue of figurative language by drawing attention to the story line of a poem. In much of lyric poetry there is often a series of images held together by either simile or metaphor; the puzzle-like nature of poetry becomes even more pronounced. It seems that the transition was a logical one, for the subdued narrator in Haiku could not deal with the personal comments that the students wanted to make. They were ready to deal with a narrator and, perhaps because of the hearing-impaired student's need for action, were not comfortable in a personae-less situation.

Another reason for the move to lyric poetry is the difficulty in finding isolated similes and metaphors in material generally. Take for instance the belabored Burns' poem:

> O, my love's like a red, red rose
> That's newly sprung in June.
> O, my love's like the melodie
> That's sweetly played in tune.
>
> As fair art thou, my bonnie lass,
> So deep in love am I.
> And I will love thee still, my dear,
> Till all the seas go dry.
>
> Till all the seas go dry, my dear.
> And the rocks melt with the sun,
> And I will love thee still, my dear.
> While the sands of life shall rune. . .

The first two stanzas are manageable; comparison of love to a rose, a sweet melodie and seas running dry. But the third stanza employs some metaphorical images which obviously could not be explained by similes and isolated metaphors. What are the possibilities of rocks melting in the sun? What is happening with the sands of life? Although this image has become cliché to us, to the young hearing-impaired reader it can be misread and trigger images of sand that is alive, racing on the beach. There are not too many dead metaphors in the hearing-impaired child's experience. He is still confined to literal interpretation. The goal should not be to have the reader try to analyze or measure the metaphoric intent of the writer but rather to see, if only partially, what the writer was seeing.

If we look at the metaphor using the accepted terminology of literary critics, the subject of the comparison is called the **tenor** and the image which communicates or carries the idea is called the **vehicle.** This schema sees the metaphor as a construct which holds variants in tension. Whether it be to extend and enhance the description or to draw that thing into a series of images, figurative language is one of the most rewarding aspects of reading literature and creative writing.

In Burns' poem a student can perhaps visualize the beach receding, or the winds blowing the sand or, as one student did, see the image of the sand clock, but how does this fit into the poem? We approached this question in part by helping the student to discover that *sand* (the vehicle) represents *time* (the tenor). The statement "And I will love thee still, my dear" becomes powerful when one realizes that love will endure the swift passage of the "sands of life."

Because of the age group I felt that contemporary music could be interesting to get into. The songs of Simon and Garfunkel seemed like a good place to begin. We began with "I Am A Rock." The two central metaphors were isolated and we discussed the qualities of both words (*rock* and *island*). The class saw the lifelessness of a rock and the solitude of an island as two things that were not like people at all. But why should the narrator be making such a statement?

Verse by verse we analyzed the setting, tone and mood. What feelings go along with winter days? How can a person be a fortress? How can this room be like a womb? The images seemed disjointed and confusing. However, the students were becoming more conscious of the parts of the poem. The descriptive significance of the words was becoming more important. The poet's use of the word *shroud*, for instance, was shown as a need on the narrator's part to emphasize the secretive, silencing nature of the snow. A discussion of defense mechanisms followed. We talked of how people protect their emotions or sometimes even destroy them; their defenses are like a fortress. All along we emphasized the power of the words chosen. We discussed what books and reading do for us; how they allow us to escape into another world. Books can be like armour. Again there is a heavy reliance on the descriptive verb *shielded*.

Basically what had to be done was to take the metaphors and break them down into more manageable similes, and then combine the images to create a tenor. Students wrote:

Snow is like a blanket.
The trees are like frozen dancers.
The smoke from the chimneys hangs over the house like clouds.

All of the above similes create a vehicle to talk about the tenor, winter. Once the students could write these simple similes, they could understand the narrator's claim to be a rock or an island.

I have found throughout my work with lyric poetry that many students are anxious to listen to the music while following along with the words. Very often I would say or sign the words at the same time. The change in rhythm in the last two lines of the song helps suggest the irony of those lines.

As a contrast to "I Am A Rock" we next did "Old Friends." In this case there is a major simile rather than a controlling metaphor. The students were responsive in offering up ideas about companionship and the needs of old people. The idea of emotional support was taken from the image of the men sitting like bookends. Again, listening to the music was a great help in talking of tone and mood. (*FIGURE 8.67*)

The second stanza posed a problem. One student suggested the sunset was death. He

---

"OLD FRIENDS"

Tenor
Old *friends*
Old *friends*
Sat on a park bench,
Vehicle
like *bookends*.
A newspaper blown through the grass
Falls on the round toes,
the high shoes,
of the Old Friends.

Old friends,
Winter companions,
the old men
Lost in their overcoats,
Waiting for the sunset.

Tenor
The sounds of the city,
Sifting through trees,
Vehicle
Settle like *dust* on the shoulders.
Of the Old friends.
Can you imagine us
Years from today
Sharing a park bench quietly?
How terribly strange to be seventy.
Old friends,
Memory brushes the same years,
Silently sharing the same fears.

FIGURE 8.67

pointed to the last line of the poem as positive proof that the theme was death. As a class we analyzed stanza two again. The students were asked to describe what they saw in their mind's eye; old men, swallowed up by overcoats, sitting on a park bench in a noisy city waiting for evening.

There were questions I had to ask. Why was the sound settling like dust? Why did the poet say "shoulders" instead of park bench or ground? Why is it winter rather than spring? In answering these questions we began forming a cluster of images into a con-

"APRIL, COME SHE WILL"

April, come she will,
When streams are ripe and swelled with rain.
May she will stay,
Resting in my arms again.
June, she'll change her tune,
In restless walks she'll prowl the night.
July, she will fly,
And give no warning to her flight.
August, die she must,
The autumn winds blow chilly and cold.
September, I'll remember
A love once new has now grown old.

FIGURE 8.68

trolling theme. The class was inadvertently isolating the tenor *time* through grasping its vehicles, sunset, and dust. Of course, sunset can be handled as a universal symbol, but isn't it more liberating to allow each individual to create his own system of symbols?

As my next selection I wanted a poem with many related images from which a tenor and a vehicle could be extracted. I had in mind something like Shakespeare's Sonnet #73, "That time of year thou mayst in me behold," with its beautiful vehicles for time, but I was sure that much more work was necessary before the students could approach this sonnet. I chose instead Simon's "April Come She Will." (*FIGURE 8.68*) By unanimous agreement the students proclaimed it a beautiful poem about seasons. One brave soul suggested that it was the story of a bird befriended by the narrator.

It was difficult to try and point students toward an alternative interpretation. They seemed so rigid at times, but to force an interpretation was disastrous. If that initial response and communion between poem and reader is constrained, poetry can become bland and lifeless. For this reason we deferred judgment on "April" and read Paul McCartney's "Eleanor Rigby" (1968), in which the meaning was more obvious to the class. The students discussed its theme in relation to the other poems they had read.

The following day we began work on "April" again. I asked the class, "If this poem is about a bird who comes to live with the narrator, can you explain the last line? Why does the love grow old?" After some floundering they determined that good love stays young and beautiful, while bad love becomes old and ugly. One student agreed that maybe the poem wasn't about a bird after all. But the class still struggled with the *flight* in July and the *prowling* in June. They could not see how these verbs functioned as metaphors for the months of the year.

Through none too subtle methods I initiated discussions about the months of the year. New love is like spring; it grows through the summer. Fall is like approaching death. Hence, love grows old like autumn leaves. By this time everyone had recognized that the poem was about lost love. In retrospect, a better way of approaching this might have been to ask the class to supply metaphors for love and love lost and then to introduce the poem itself.

Using the metaphor in this poem, we were able to construct our own similes and metaphors.

In April streams are like ripe fruit.
In June love is like a singing bird.
Then love walks like a cat.
Love is like a bird. It flies away
In August, love dies like the leaves and
flowers because summer is ending.

The vehicles are all of these, the tenor is love. We could now talk about *rock* and *island* in analytical terms.

"I AM A ROCK."

I–tenor
rock, island–vehicles which carry thoughts of death and isolation.

Another Simon poem which I thought the class might be able to understand was "Bridge Over Troubled Water." I was surprised at the difficulty we encountered. The major simile was very confusing for the class. ". . . like a bridge over troubled water, I will lay me down." They could evaluate the properties of a bridge to go as far as stating "I will be like a bridge," but they were troubled by the physical impossibility of such a statement. They were not interpreting *troubled water* adequately. This problem obscured the entire meaning of the poem for them. We listed those images which we saw before us; weariness, feeling small, tears in your eyes, rough times, evening falling hard, pain all around. These images expressed the sorrows, defeats and pains of life. The students were then asked to write simple similes or metaphors taken from the poem. The results:

Darkness is troubled waters.
Times get rough like troubled waters.
Tears are like troubled waters.
Comfort is like a bridge.
Friends are like bridges over troubled water.

The vehicle *troubled water* became synonymous for problems in life. The tenor *I* remained constant: I will always be right behind you.

Previously we had compared Haiku to simple declarative remarks. I was curious as to whether the students could see the advantages of sometimes using metaphorical language in everyday description. They were asked to choose which statement had more meaning for them:

I will be helpful when you are depressed.
or
I will be your bridge over troubled water.

Honestly, two students preferred the literal statement.

By identifying the tenor and vehicle within an image a structural framework for organizing metaphorical language was provided for the students. They then analyzed their own metaphors.

1. The maple leaves are shooting stars.
   When they shake,
   fireworks
   explode.

   tenor–*leaves in autumn*
   vehicle–*stars and fireworks,* (shimmering colors)

2. The raindrops crawled down the stem.
   tenor–*raindrop*
   vehicle-*things that crawl* (allusion to insects)

3. Rain is falling on tall skeletons with no gloves.
   Arms vibrating.
   tenor–*trees in winter*
   vehicle–*skeleton, branches* (allusion to dead things)

It is important to point out that we should not try to force a specific interpretation on the students but rather show them that isolating things, like tenor and vehicle, can be of great help in understanding metaphorical language. Some students will cling to similes. "The ocean was like thousands of hills." "I saw the sky with clouds which were covering it like a tent." I think that more complex metaphorical language will follow once they begin to see and think in metaphors. For some it is still a very contrived and difficult process, but figurative language pricks the imagination, forcing us to look more closely at life. Without it the imagination can lay dormant and wither and we remain prisoners and victims of literal interpretation.

They See, You See, I See: Art, An Experience To Learn

by Peter J. Geisser

Millions of tiny fragments of broken dreams are brought together in a place of learning.
And because men and women take the time-
Silent children sing and hear the music which sets souls dancing.
Millions of tiny fragments are brought together and what was broken, with years of patient learning, becomes whole again,
And a new world emerges filled with broken children made whole!

I am an artist who teaches. I taught hearing students at the Museum of Fine Arts in Boston for many years and at another school for the deaf for three years. I married a teacher of the hearing-impaired and through her incredible commitment I became committed to the education of the hearing-impaired myself.

In my first year at the Rhode Island School for the Deaf the art program focused on the needs of the lower and middle schools. The development of skills in the younger children is essential for a good art program, but as important and so often neglected is the development of cultural awareness through the exposure to and the relevance of the fine arts. It is my observation that, contrary to popular platitudes, hearing-impaired children do not see better than hearing children. In fact, I find the language difficulties that hearing-impaired children have seriously affected their perception and creativity.

The middle school was studying units on the Middle Ages, the Renaissance and the Age of Exploration. The school was, at that time, small enough to introduce my theory that art could be a unifying factor in the total curriculum design. The students were amazed that the man in the art room knew what they were learning in English and social studies. This interdisciplinary approach was enriching, not only for the students but also for the faculty because the students were building relationships between the various subject areas. Chaucer's pilgrims were part of a feudal system which produced the Canterbury Cathedral. Chaucer was studied in the language class, the feudal system in social studies and the Cathedral in art.

In my second year at the Rhode Island School for the Deaf the school was in the process of moving to our present facility at Corliss Park. The high school was separated

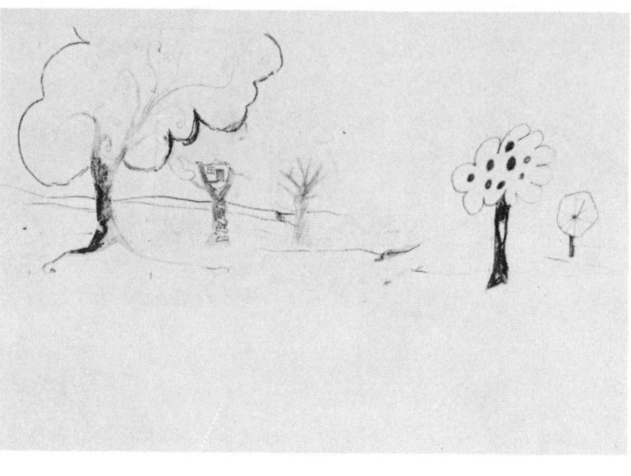

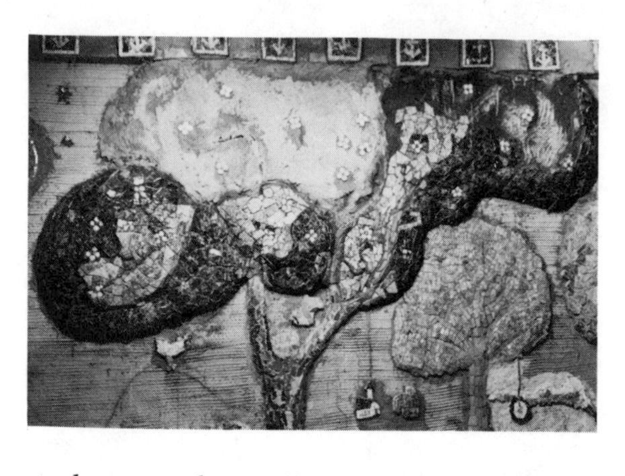

FIGURE 8.69 A twenty-five foot mosaic mural was fashioned from over three hundred children's drawings

from the rest of the school in the move and the morale was at an ebb. We needed something to pull the tremendous energies working at the school together in some basic direction while the trauma of relocation passed. The art program aimed itself at creating a great work of art.

Drawings were made by all of the children, from 2 to 20 years of age. *(FIGURE 8.69)* For several weeks I played the part of visual conductor, pulling over three hundred drawings into an idyllic landscape which would become a 25-foot mosaic mural for the lobby of the new school. Every person in the school participated in some way; every art class was in some way working on it.

Happily, everyone was talking about the work that was coming to life as well as the headaches of moving. Language classes were writing about the mural, science classes were taking trips to the wall to see how the mortar was made, and math and social studies classes studied graphs, maps, scale models and how to enlarge things from scale. At one point the contractor said we could begin assembling the mosaic on the wall as long as it was after 5 p.m. when the workmen were not there! We cancelled all but the lower school art classes and I worked a night shift with a couple of the older students so that we could complete the mosaic. Rudy, a middle school student, made it all worthwhile when he came in one morning and told me, "It was like Michaelangelo and Pope July, you know Mr. Geisser, work all night and just get bother, bother, bother." Rudy had made the connection. A year before he had learned about the Renaissance and the frustration which Michaelangelo endured under his patron Pope Julius II while creating the Sistine Chapel frescoes. The process of producing a monumental work of art gave reality to what had been studied. The exposure had been internalized but it wasn't something that would have shown up on a test. The five trees in the mural, which are a visual pun on the Rhode Island curriculum, show the five distinct levels of language development. But that such a mural should be created as part of the school's art and language program shows a far more significant development in the field of education of the hearing impaired.

The mural had proven that art could, in fact, be the language that all levels of hearing-impaired children could understand, participate in and truly be native speakers of. The timing according to the development of the Rhode Island curriculum was ripe and the high school was coming of age. We offered the senior art program to the class of 1976.

The purpose of the course was to show that men of all times have found the means to express their ephemeral being in material symbols. In a letter to parents explaining this program I wrote:

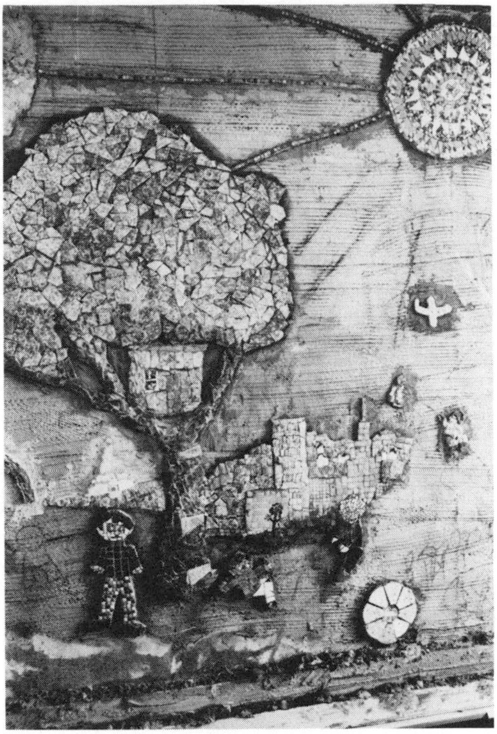

FIGURE 8.70 Science, math and social studies used the mural to teach skills in measurement and mapping.

"I have been teaching art to the deaf for six years. In this time I have seen the need for the arts to become a part of every deaf person's life; very much the same way that music is a part of every hearing person's life, whether it's Beethoven on a stereo or hard rock on the way to work. At the end of this year I hope our seniors will see that the harmony which Beethoven wrote and never heard is the same harmony that happens in dance, in a basketball game, and in painting!"

The text for the course is Janson's History of Art for Young People (1971). The students were asked not to read any of the book until they had enough knowledge from the class presentation to handle its language and context. There is nothing like a prohibition to stimulate interest in a book. By midterm many of the students had read the entire book!

Rather than starting with the cave man and giving a name and date to every work of art and author up to the present day, I chose to develop the categorization process (which can be so poor in hearing-impaired students) as well as to develop the process of generalization. Thus, the prehistoric period was typified in the symbol of Earth Mother; the Egyptians in their quest for eternity; the Greeks in their search for perfection; the Romans in their acquisition of power; the Middle Ages as the quest for heaven; the Renaissance as the search for identity; and the present day as the amalgamation of all times.

At the beginning of the year, while presenting the symbolic level of art, the school's principal Peter Blackwell presented a comparison of creation myths to the class. The reoccurrence of clay as a symbol lead to a whole lesson on hidden meaning and metaphor. Creativity can be defined as the ability to make metaphor; to put unlike things together in a way that they communicate, be these things visual or verbal. Creativity is a language functioning.

One of the middle school classes with a low language level was doing a poem about creation so I did the same presentation with this class. The results still haunt me.

I had a lump of clay which we labeled as *dead*. The second lump of clay I made into a pot "before your very eyes" and we labeled it as *alive*. We called the pot a vessel and discussed all the things a vessel could do; hold water, hold flowers, hold milk. I then took a finished pot filled with water and broke it. The vessel was alive; the broken vessel was dead (and Mr. Geisser was labeled as a "bad boy"). We talked about grinding up the broken pot and making it into clay again. This related to the life's cycle which the students had learned in another class. Then the great metaphor came. I wrote, "Home from school every Joan day goes." Everyone agreed that my language was bad. Then I wrote "Joan goes home from school everyday." We saw that the first sentence was just words while the other was a sentence with good language. Joan, who related to my sentence more than the other kids, said "Clay dead, vessel alive; words dead, language alive." What more was there to learn?

Perhaps the most valuable thing that spun out of the senior art program is the interdisciplinary learning that has begun at the school. This year the seniors are offered a literature course which parallels the art program. The juniors are taking Western Civilization which prepares them for the art program.

At about the end of the Renaissance presentations I showed the group a portrait of Frans Hals, the famous 17th century Dutch painter. Manny's eyes lit up. He exclaimed, "These people look like they are the same time as William Shakespeare." We found the painting was painted in 1025. "They look like the pilgrims. Pilgrims came to America in 1620! The Pilgrims lived in Holland for a time before they came to America!" One painting brought the search for identity, which we called the Renaissance, into focus for Manny. The Pilgrims were not related to the studies of Leonardo DaVinci but now, because of seeing the Pilgrims as part of the Renaissance, many isolated bits of knowledge became integrated and internalized.

The seniors were having difficulty with various concepts, such as abstraction, metaphor, categorization and generalization, so we presented these concepts to younger children in an attempt to broaden the curriculum at its base. The lower school was doing a unit on the ancient Greeks. The classroom teacher had taught the students that the Greeks had many gods, and compared their religion with the Judeo-Christian religions of today which have only one god. When the class came to art we looked at the Christian churches and Greek temples. As a project we drew a mural of Athens with all its ancient temples. When it was just about time to go back to class, 8-year-old David took a marker and put crosses on the tops of all the Greek temples. "Us one God, Greeks many gods!" David had the concept of monotheism and polytheism. He also said, "Us churches; Greeks temples."

A visitor to the school asked if this error was then corrected. Thinking I must be missing something I asked "What error?" "Well, the objective of the lesson was to have the student understand the difference between monotheism and polytheism, but if he believes that Greek temples have crosses he clearly hasn't met the objective." This is where I smile at the behavioral objectives and take "behavioral objection." In a spiral developmental approach to learning, it is quite kosher to put crosses on temples if, as in David's case, those crosses are the symbols that say "Greeks many, many gods."

David is 8 years old and at this age it is far more important to understand the concept than the specific fact. In a few years David will again encounter ancient Greece and will bring to it an understanding that can be developed, rather than facts to be corrected.

In an exam on Egyptian art I gave the seniors this question:

In Egyptian history, there were three main periods of time:

the Old Kingdom
the Middle Kingdom
the New Kingdom

a) Which period did Mycerinus live in?
b) Which period did Nefertiti come from?

Mycerinus live in Egypt.
Nefertiti come from Egypt.
The Old Kingdom was first develop relative of God and very strick rule and power.
The Middle Kingdom was more powerful then Old Kingdom and more freedom and more art.
The New Kingdom was more powerful but Egyptian became boring rule and fall (apart).

Denise typified the problem of testing for facts vs. concepts by answering that Mycerinus lived in Egypt; Nefertiti came from Egypt. These were good answers from any hearing-impaired person brought up on the

Fitzgerald Key – a preposition needs an object – Egypt is a noun. Happily, Denise continued her answer describing the three periods of Egyptian art and how each evolved and influenced the other. The language difficulties got in the way of the "correct" answer, but the grammatically "correct" answer would not really show that Denise had a great understanding of the subject.

The senior class of 1976 decided not to leave the school with a traditional gift but asked my help in creating a work of art to leave the school. They illustrated the John Denver song "Looking For Space" on the walls of the school snack bar. *(FIGURE 8.71)* They also executed a stained glass mural depicting six major periods of man's history. This group of students, through their hard work, also proved that cultural awareness for hearing-impaired students is a must.

The senior art program worked. It has opened opportunities to all our students to integrate their entire school experience with the help of the language of art. Thanks to Mr. Don Gardner of the State Department of Education, we have three hearing students taking the senior art program with six hearing-impaired students this year. We have reverse integration. While studying the history of visual communication these students are experiencing their own history of communication, comparing their life experiences not only to the Pharoahs, but also to each other.

Last week the seniors–hearing and hearing-impaired–brought a class of 7-year-olds to the Rhode Island School of Design museum. Dorothy, one of our seniors, reflected on the trip:

"Three hearing students and senior class went to RISD Museum with lower school kids. Suzanne was with me as I was teaching and showing her some of Rome big stone. Suzanne arrived at the stone. She said, 'The angel's body seems strong and fat faces.' I was explaining to Suzanne about the man from the Middle Ages whose sign with the

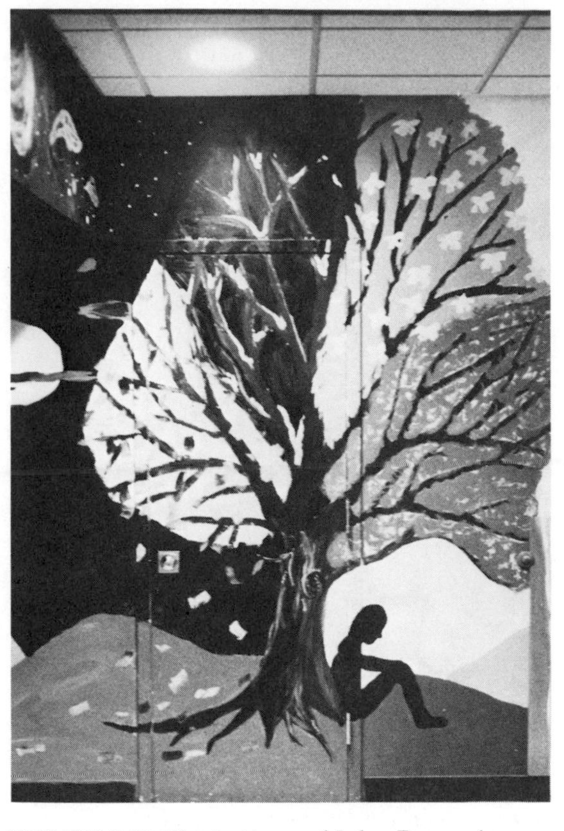

FIGURE 8.71 Illustrations of John Denver's song "Looking for Space" decorate the walls of the school snack bar

hands said 'wonderful and wow.' Suzanne said, 'Oh, he is deaf!' I laughed. . .

"I feel that Suzanne and other kids who are just like me as I was small. They arrived and stared as things at RISD Museum. I compare to me. I couldn't believe that I was growing, right now, I have a new experience which I'll finish my school with." On the way home from the museum, Mathew, a hearing student petrified of young deaf children, proudly proclaimed: "We understood each other! I never thought little kids could see so much!" Quite frankly, neither did I.

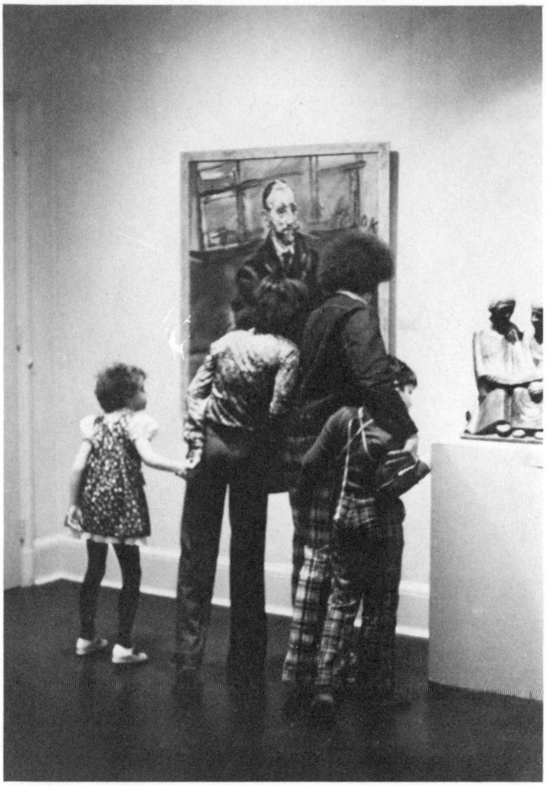

"One time, Peter showed us one slide named 'Guernica' made by Pablo Picasso. We can't imagine how big it was. So when we got there, our mouth opened very widely because it was really huge in about a full one side of a room.

"We walked to St. Patrick's Cathedral across from Museum of Modern Art. We stopped and looked outside the Cathedral. WOW! Hard to believe because a long time ago this Cathedral was the tallest building in N. Y. City area, but right now the many tall buildings stood around the Cathedral. Poor Cathedral!

"On the way [home] we talked about this day which we enjoyed. We fell asleep because our eyes were very tired of looking [at] many new things all day. One thing I said 'Good Bye' to New York City when we were on route 95. We got at RISD at 3:00 a.m. I don't care how late it was and how tired I was because I really enjoyed the day which I will never forget."

Nancy Vinacco

"I really wanted to touch on things of museum, but the sign said, 'Do not touch.' Because I wanted to know feelings [of the] past in the Middle Ages."

Hansell Germond

"What is art? What is Art's life? You can do and learn. Everyone can, too. Everyone can build in the future. Everyone can imagine, create, work. . . and do anything. My senior art program class can learn, experience, and can build ourselves for the future. We can feel anything in the arts . . . You can make creative the arts and [everything]. We can feel deeply through [everything]. We can love and dislike anything. We enjoy to learn the arts now and in the future."

Gary Fortier

When Peter showed me slides of the palaces, courtyards, gates and buildings, I tried to imagine that I was in France. The slides gave me a little idea and feeling. But we went to Brown University campus, and walked through the tunnel into the beautiful atmosphere. As I stood in the middle of land surrounding buildings, I couldn't believe that it was like the palace. I was completely inside the small world blocking out the city. Greek, Roman, Gothic, and modern buildings (were) around me and (I) felt like I (was) living through all the periods of time. It gave me the feelings of importance. If I didn't learn anything about Art, I would probably miss the beauty in life. I couldn't believe myself that I learned so much but I just couldn't express myself.

Lena Ferro

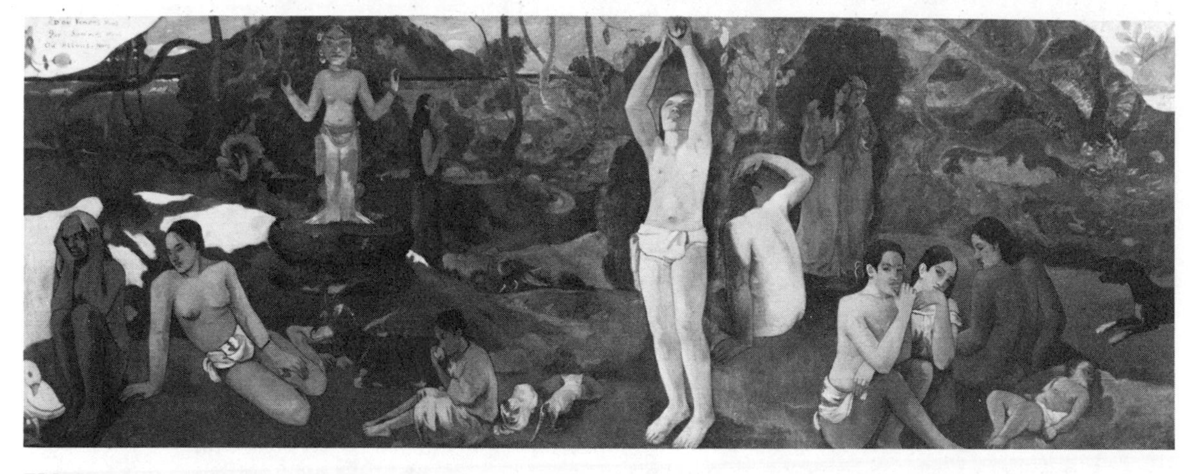

FIGURE 8.73 "D' ou Venons-Nous. . . Que Sommes-Nous . . . Ou Allons-Nous?" (Where have we come from?) by Paul Gauguin

When I went into the Boston Museum of fine Arts, I looked at the painting. Wow! I felt greatly involved in this painting and I saw a lot of expression and I felt completely knowledgable about the painting. I never had this feeling before. I felt the most expression with Gauguin's painting which is (Where are they come from, What are we doing, where are we going?) the slide of this painting was not a complete expression to me and I thought, it was not realy pretty. But when I saw real this painting, then it was a beautiful expression to me.

When my eyes looked at the expresstionism painting, It amazed me. I felt like I was moving, for example I feel like a wave, like peace, like spot, like pep, like smooth, like wild, and many different moving things. And I feel like I was in the painting. I hated to leave each Art room and finally I hated to leave this Museum.

Then we had to leave. Our eyes became tired. It was time to pull our eye's blinds down to rest.

Denise James

ACKNOWLEDGMENTS

FIGURES

Page 128 *Figure 8.59* From unit prepared by Charles Girard, Rhode Island School for the Deaf.

Page 131 *Figure 8.60,* Page 131 *Figure 8.61,* Page 133 *Figure 8.62,* Page 135 *Figure 8.63,* Page 136 *Figure 8.64,* Page 137 *Figure 8.65* From unit prepared by Jeffrey R. Cole and Judith Gilman Garland, Rhode Island School for the Deaf.

Page 137 *Figure 8.66* Photograph courtesy of Ira Garber.

Page 140 *Figure 8.67* "Old Friends" by Paul Simon. Copyright © 1968 by Paul Simon. Reprinted by permission of the author.

Page 141 *Figure 8.68* From "April, Come She Will" by Paul Simon. Copyright © 1965 by Paul Simon. Reprinted by permission of the author.

Page 144 *Figure 8.69,* Page 145 *Figure 8.70* Photographs courtesy of Peter Geisser. Drawings and murals by the students under the supervision of Peter Geisser, Rhode Island School for the Deaf.

Page 147 *Figure 8.71* Photograph courtesy of Ira Garber. Mural by senior class, Rhode Island School for the Deaf.

Page 149 *Figure 8.73* "D'ou Venons-Nous . . . Que Sommes-Nous . . . Ou Allons-Nous?" by Paul Gauguin, canvas. Tompkins Gallery, courtesy of Museum of Fine Arts, Boston.

Chapter 9

Language Assessment

Goals of a Language Evaluation

The question often asked by teachers of the hearing impaired is, "How do I know where to start in teaching language?" or "How do I know what my students need?" In many schools for the hearing impaired there is no linguist or language specialist to help the teacher with the task of language assessment. It thus becomes the classroom teacher's responsibility to evaluate the linguistic level of her students and to set language goals.

The purpose of this chapter is to outline in broad terms an approach to language assessment that could be used by a classroom teacher or by the teacher and a specialist in collaboration. The first section discusses the categories to be considered in such an assessment and the background for the approach described here. The second section describes the collection of linguistic data used in assessing the comprehension and production of language and some of the problems involved in language sampling. A third section describes specific tools used in evaluation, both formal and informal, and the advantages and disadvantages of various techniques used in assessment. The final section discusses how to evaluate the results of this testing and data collection. Examples from actual language evaluations are used throughout to illustrate and clarify the discussion.

The general objective of an evaluation of this kind is to describe the student's level of linguistic functioning, competence as well as performance, so the teacher can build on that competence and proceed in an organized and productive manner toward the next level. To achieve this objective one should evaluate both comprehension and production since an evaluation based solely on production provides an incomplete picture of the child's competence. The relationship between comprehension and production helps to reveal the child's progress in language acquisition.

The specific goal is to evaluate the child's comprehension, production and use of language, however delayed or minimal it may be, in terms of what it indicates about his progress toward a complete language system. There are many measures which could be used to describe a student's linguistic functioning. Among these are length of utterance, frequency of usage of the various parts of speech, development of morphology, and such specific measures as the ratio of nouns to verbs. The continuum described in this book, however, which outlines 1) the prerequisites for language acquisition, 2) the simple sentence level and 3) the acquisition of complex structures, can provide a useful and relevant scale for describing progress in language acquisition.

One aspect of a language evaluation, then, is to determine where the student is on this scale. Does his expressive language, for instance, consist of one-word utterances or some limited connected language? Can he reliably produce simple sentences and perhaps attempt some complex sentences? Even this level of assessment gives the teacher a place to start in planning language work. Knowing that the student has a good grasp of simple sentences allows her to plan language work to further refine the use of simple sentences (with attention to the syntactical and semantic considerations outlined in Chapter 5) as well as to plan controlled exposure to the complex structures that will comprise the next stage of language acquisition.

Attaining a level of linguistic development is not an all-or-nothing affair. It is not like becoming 10 years old, acquiring a new tooth or learning to ride a bicycle. A child does not suddenly reach a stage where he magically produces good simple sentences and never again an incomplete or faulty one. One can only observe that the child seems to be at a simple sentence stage because the majority of his utterances demonstrate this. He may still demonstrate a reversion to telegraphic or truncated utterances in certain situations or seem to be in several stages simultaneously.

It is more productive to use what is known about the acquisition of language structure as a standard of comparison rather than to compare children according to some inappropriate criteria. Although there are some parameters which are useful in the evaluation process, there are many which are not. For example, comparison by chronological age – how far the child is from being on a par with his age group linguistically – is not particularly relevant in evaluating hearing-impaired children. There are many factors that influence progress more than simply chronological age, such as etiology, age of onset of loss, type of loss, age of discovery of loss, and the crucial factor of parental support.

Age does become an important consideration, however, when the evaluation has been completed and recommendations for language work are made. The conceptual basis and content material used to accomplish language goals would be very different for the 7-year-old student who does not have a simple sentence grammar, for instance, than for a 14-year-old at the same level. And although it is important to utilize what is known about acquisition of language by the "normal" child, one must be cautious about using tests which are constructed for and normed on hearing children. In many cases these tests do not provide a good basis for comparison since the hearing-impaired child may acquire language at a slower rate and possibly in a different developmental sequence.

For example, it is predictable that the function words and grammatical morphemes of Stage II language (Brown, 1973) in the hearing child will be acquired much later by the hearing-impaired child. But the important question is how this affects the child's further development. How does the fact that the hearing-impaired child functions through a long period of his language development with primarily content words affect the development that does take place, both cognitively and linguistically? One must also ask whether it is fair to assume that the hearing-impaired child is communicating the same kind of meaning with his one word as a hearing child is at the same stage, since he comes to this stage later and remains in it for a longer period of time.

These are the kinds of questions one must consider and it is for these reasons that measuring a hearing-impaired child's acquisition of language solely against norms developed for hearing children is not sufficient. Overall, the important point is not how the child compares with other children (with or without normal hearing) but where he is on the developmental continuum at the time of assessment.

Whatever the purpose of a language evaluation, it should take into consideration the child's total environment and relate language behavior to nonlanguage behavior. While we are not primarily interested in assigning diagnostic labels that sometimes can be more detrimental than helpful, it would be foolish to ignore signs that point to other problems that interfere with the acquisition of language. Sociolinguistic and psychological aspects of language behavior must be considered, as well as other handicapping conditions that will affect the child's progress.

Consideration of the child's home situation and home language is, of course, an important factor in assessing progress and in planning an educational program. In some parts of the country, hearing-impaired children from non-English-speaking homes are placed in programs where they are expected to learn English at a stage in their development when they are not yet able to discriminate between the school language and the home language. During a recent evaluation it was discovered that a 7-year-old child actually was exposed to three languages in his environment; English at school and a combination of Portuguese and Creole (the dialect of the Cape Verdes islands) at home.

Another consideration is the quality of the communication between child, parents and siblings. The most basic question is whether the parents attempt to communicate with the child and in what mode. The relationship between modes of communication comes into consideration here, as well as the attitude of the family toward using various modes. One evaluation revealed that in a family consisting of hearing parents, two hearing-impaired children and two hearing children, the hearing-impaired children used their manual communication to reject those members of the family who did not understand sign language. Manipulating language modes in this way will influence the child's attitude and motivation for achieving in an oral classroom.

Since the goal is to evaluate linguistic competence, the assessment should be conducted in any and all modes used by the child to produce language. The observational techniques, tests and methods described herein can be utilized in assessing oral language, sign language, written language or any combination thereof. Sampling the student's linguistic behavior in a variety of situations and settings is essential for achieving a balanced and realistic assessment. Data from objective measures, language behavior with family, peers and strangers, and response to classroom materials and activities should all be included to achieve as complete a picture as possible. In fact, if setting language goals is the objective, observation of the student's behavior in the classroom may actually be more important than the results of formal testing. The classroom situation provides observation of the child when he is comfortable and actively engaged in communication.

The end result of the language evaluation proposed here is a description in narrative form of the student's linguistic functioning. It should present a realistic assessment of what he understands, what he can reliably express and how he uses his language; that is, comprehension, production and function – a language profile rather than a collection of test scores. Although it is not necessary to describe performance in numerical terms to achieve a language profile, scores of this type can also be useful and relevant, particularly in collecting and developing in-house norms. The approach to assessment delineated here utilizes broad categories rather than overly detailed scoring systems. Hopefully this approach avoids the pitfalls of rigid assessment procedures which lead to lock-step developmental schemes.

Assessment of Production and Comprehension

This section discusses the various aspects of language to be considered in evaluation, beginning with a discussion of data collection for evaluating language production (expressive language).

In analyzing and describing a child's expressive language, one should sample his spontaneous language in a variety of situations as a means of assessing both linguistic performance and competence. An extensive sample of what is actually expressed (performance) is necessary in order to learn something about the underlying system of rules (competence). The problem with this dichotomy is that, while linguistic performance is available to record and analyze, the child's linguistic competence must be inferred from this performance. The question becomes how much one can rely on inference for information about linguistic competence. This is particularly a problem in assessing the language of hearing-impaired children since there is often so much missing from their language performance. As stated earlier, it is imperative that the competence/performance distinction be kept in mind and that the child's ability is not underestimated on the basis of his possibly poor performance.

Performance can be affected by many factors such as fatigue, motivation and the child's feeling about which communication style is called for by the situation. In the case of hearing-impaired children, some may use predominantly telegraphic language when communicating with other children but be capable of using standard English when the situation demands it. Another child may only be capable of a telegraphic production. One aspect of an evaluation might then be to judge the appropriateness of a child's communication style to the situation.

Another problem confronting the evaluator is how to interpret telegraphic language. For instance, given the following sample of spontaneous oral language of a 6-year-old child, what conclusions can be reached about her acquisition of simple sentences? (*FIGURE 9.74*) When a child produces utterances of the type of #s 6, 12, 13, 14, and 15, do we conclude that she is producing a pattern three sentence with the verb *to be* omitted? Or is this type of utterance a noun phrase with nonstandard word order? Do we credit her with a sentence structure or a phrase structure? It might be useful to look at the hearing child's development in a case such as this. If hearing children produce similar omissions we might conclude that this child's language is not deviant but delayed.

Unfortunately there are no easy answers to these questions. Arriving at a reasonable conclusion becomes easier with a larger sample of utterances. With a sample large enough to include the distribution and usage of the utterances in *FIGURE 9.74* it might be possible to draw some conclusions about this child's acquisition of sentence structures.

Spontaneous Oral Language From a Six-Year-Old Hearing-Impaired Child

1. I forgot.
2. Not now.
3. Father no work finish.
4. My father finish.
5. Mary cry outside.
6. Boy bad.
7. Mary play.
8. Miss Sue far away.
9. Joan eat.
10. Joan paint.
11. Before paint remember?
12. Mary bad boot.
13. Sad Joan
14. Different chair.
15. Dark house.
16. Hair cut.
17. Tomorrow birthday father.
18. I want juice.
19. I want paper towel.
20. Sit down watch.

FIGURE 9.74 Sample of spontaneous oral language from a six-year-old severely to profoundly hearing-impaired child.

COLLECTION OF LANGUAGE SAMPLES

As stated previously, to collect a language sample representative of the child's language and linguistic functioning, data should be gathered from as many different situations with as many different people as possible. One wants to know what kind of language the child produces in response to questions, both in the structured context of the classroom and in the testing situation devoid of helpful environmental and contextual clues; one wants to determine how he communicates with his peers, how he communicates with his siblings and parents, and how he communicates with adults other than those he is familiar with.

This last type of data might be the most important of all and is a strong argument for having someone with whom the child is not particularly familiar conduct at least a part of

RESPONSES TO QUESTIONS

QUESTION	RIGHT CATEGORY	WRONG CATEGORY
Where does the boy live?	Texas	cow
What does the boy have?	horse	small
Who is riding the horse?	boy	far away
Why are they putting food there?	to eat	cow, food
Where are they sitting?	restaurant	watch

FIGURE 9.75 *Examples of answers in the right category illustrating that the question form was understood and examples of answers in the wrong category.*

the evaluation. The reasons for this are described succinctly by Brown (1973) in his conclusions about the linguistic functioning of the hearing child in Stage II.

"In Stage II and after we shall see that he operates, often for long periods, as if grammatical morphemes were optional. Furthermore, the child's omissions are by no means limited to the relatively lawful omissions which also often occur in adult speech. He often leaves out what is linguistically obligatory. This suggests to me that the child expects always to be understood if he produces any appropriate words at all. And in fact we find that he would usually be right in this expectation as long as he speaks at home, in familiar surroundings, and to family members who know his history and inclinations. Stage I speech may then be said to be well adapted to its communicative purpose, well adapted but narrowly adapted. In new surroundings and with less familiar addressees it would often fail. This suggests that a major dimension of linguistic development is learning to express always and automatically certain things (agent, action, number, tense and so on) even though these meanings may be in many particular contexts quite redundant. The child who is going to move out into the world, as children do, must learn to make his speech broadly and flexibly adaptive" (p. 245).

These observations are as pertinent to the development of the hearing-impaired child as to that of the hearing child. In a school for the hearing-impaired it is common to overhear a young child relate an incident using minimal sentence structure and nearly unintelligible speech and yet be perfectly understood by the teacher. Communication takes place because the teacher "knows the child's history and inclinations" and essentially already knows the story. The child, therefore, is very narrowly adapted, being understood by his family and teachers but not by the world. And so it is tremendously important that one evaluates how the child is progressing in terms of making his speech broadly and flexibly adaptive to any situation.

Aside from this aspect of data sampling, the teacher is in the advantageous position of being able to collect language samples over a period of time. Essentially every time she asks a question in class she has the opportunity to evaluate the child's ability to respond to question forms as well as to the content and ideas presented in the material. Given a well-defined idea of what she is asking from the child (whether she is interested in answers per se, responses to certain types of question forms or the structure of the response itself), the teacher can evaluate particular aspects of the child's linguistic ability. She must always be cognizant, however, that her familiarity with the child and the material does not cause her to overinterpret the child's answers. Certainly the teacher is in the best position to know with what material the child is familiar and this should enable her to decide what a wrong answer signals. Perhaps the question form was not understood or the vocabulary was unfamiliar, or the child understood the question but simply did not know the answer. *(FIGURE 9.75)*

The teacher is also in a good position to sample the child's ability to **ask** questions. This is an aspect of language evaluation often neglected because of the difficulty in eliciting it from the child. Classroom practices require the child to answer questions much more often than to ask them, and for many hearing-impaired children question formation is an area of real difficulty. While most hearing-impaired children seem to have the conceptual category of the interrogative, their ability to express questions in the appropriate syntactic form may be very limited. For instance, it is very common for a child to ask "What is your name?" by saying or signing the word "name?" along with an interrogative facial expression rather than by using the question form.

One reason for not describing a child's linguistic competence on the basis of his spontaneous language alone is that some linguistic structures occur very rarely in children's spontaneous language. For example, the passive structure, relative clauses and certainly nominalized structures are rarely used spontaneously by children and yet they are structures one would like to sample in the language of a child who is developing complex language. These structures are commonly used in written language and in adult standard English. It is often the case, particularly with a child with limited language, that an interview situation designed to collect language data actually results in a question/answer format; the interviewer asks questions and the child responds with one word answers or with short phrases. To avoid such a situation one must set up structured (and thereby somewhat unnatural) situations for the purpose of eliciting these structures. In other words, language tests must be used.

What constitutes a reasonable language sample from which to draw conclusions depends on the stated goal of the language analysis. Researchers in the field of child language, for example, want to write a complete grammar of a child's linguistic competence. They therefore feel the need to collect (by our standards) enormously large samples. Since teachers and other professionals working in a school setting have the day-to-day business of educating children, they usually have to be content with less extensive language sampling. Also, for the purposes of developing language goals and placing children in reasonable class situations, it is not necessary to be concerned with writing a grammar for each child evaluated. Therefore, a collection of around 100 utterances is reasonable to work with as long as the language is sampled in a variety of situations. A sample of this size can be collected in a short time with the aid of a good tape recorder.

Crystal et al. (1976) measure samples in terms of time rather than in terms of number of utterances and recommend using samples of thirty-minutes duration. Samples are collected in two fifteen-minute segments, the first in an unstructured free-play situation using toys as a catalyst and the second in a dialogue situation where the topic is some aspect of the child's experience. (This approach would have to be adjusted according to the child's age.) It is important that the method of collecting and analyzing language be standardized within at least one school setting so the children are evaluated and placed according to some consistent criteria.

The actual transcription of linguistic data poses problems as well. Regardless of how the sample is collected, there are certain difficulties encountered in transcribing into written form what the child expressed orally or manually. The problem may stem from trying to determine whether the child is producing connected multiword utterances or a string of one-word utterances. Because of the possible lack of intonational clues it is sometimes difficult to determine what is an utter-

SPONTANEOUS ORAL PRODUCTIONS SHOWING DIFFICULTY IN SEGMENTING

The following utterances were mostly produced without sentence intonation and in one- to three-word breath control groups. It is not always possible to distinguish between one or two word *ideas* and phrases. In this sample, commas are used to indicate the word groupings.

1. The boy asleep.
2. The dog heard.
3. Somebody throw.
4. Boy window jump, wall, foot.
5. Dirty, step, wall.
6. Big foot, bear.
7. Maybe bicycle, fall.
8. Somebody hurt, carry, go hospital, bring, hurry.
9. Outside bicycle, bicycle fall.
10. Police call, go out, carry.
11. Police call, mother come, come to hospital.
12. Man walk, car stop.
13. Dog run.
14. Fall over, orange.
15. Stop, fall over.
16. I think dog pushed.
17. Girl boy move, out of the way.
18. Street, country.
19. Maybe accident.
20. All the way.

FIGURE 9.76 Sample of spontaneous oral language illustrating the difficulty of segmenting utterances.

ance and what is a one-word idea. (*FIGURE 9.76*) The tendency of the transcriber to fill in or add intentions that were not actually present in the speaker's utterance must also be controlled. For instance, when oral (or signed) language is written down it is very easy to include punctuation and morphological endings which impart tense, plurality, phrasing and sentence contours omitted by the child. It is difficult but necessary for the transcriber to literally represent the child's output without filtering the child's language through his own linguistic system.

ASSESSMENT OF LANGUAGE COMPREHENSION

As described in Chapter 4, although the hearing child enters school with a fairly complete language system, the hearing-impaired child may have virtually no expressive language at this same age. Since expressive language (particularly oral language) develops so much more slowly in the hearing-impaired child, it is important to evaluate how comprehension of language is developing during this period.

One may be frequently faced with assessing the language of children with extremely impoverished expressive linguistic systems. Obviously it would not be very revealing or descriptive to report that the child has no language and not to evaluate further. And even when the child has some expressive language, the assessment of comprehension is imperative for a full view of the child's language ability.

Later, when connected language has begun to develop, the assessment of comprehension becomes very important in determining the relationship between receptive and expressive abilities. At this point one wants to know if the child is processing the syntax of the language he hears, even though he is not consistently showing evidence of syntax in his expressive language. In this situation, a realistic insightful evaluation of the child's comprehension can be very valuable in shedding light on his cognitive development and in determining what kind of linguistic input he will be able to utilize in building his expressive language.

The problem of assessing language comprehension raises questions which warrant some discussion. It is difficult to consider comprehension and production of language separately since the two processes are so closely tied and presumably develop hand-in-hand. Is it realistic, therefore, to consider comprehension as an isolated category of linguistic functioning? While it is generally assumed that comprehension precedes production in the hearing child, there is not much information available on the development of comprehension in the hearing-impaired child or the relationship between cognitive development and comprehension of language.

Lois Bloom (1974) presents an excellent discussion of the study of comprehension. She feels that comprehension has been largely ignored, not because its importance is not recognized but because of the difficulties in measuring it. One of the major problems is that responses involving comprehension are multidetermined; the child depends on many things besides what he hears to arrive at an understanding of an utterance. This problem is aptly illustrated by Courtney Cazden (1972).

". . . even if certain behaviors are present, the natural situation is not usually sufficiently controlled so that inferences about the child's knowledge can be made. If the adult says 'Please bring me the napkins from the kitchen table' and the child correctly brings two napkins, one cannot conclude that the child attended to and understood the meaing of the plural -s. He may have been responding simply to the presence of two napkins on the table and seen no reason to leave one behind" (p. 249).

In fact, in the case of the hearing-impaired child, he may have understood ". . . bring . . . napkin . . . kitchen" and inferred everything else from situational cues. In this case one could conclude that the child understood that an imperative requires an active response, but one cannot conclude that he understood plurals or locatives. A formal test situation, which presents structures in a contrastive situation and which forces the child to attend to a minimal difference (such as a plural morpheme) in order to respond correctly, provides much better evidence of pure linguistic processing. Sentences such as "The dogs *run*" versus "The dog *runs*," would present a true contrastive situation.

Hearing children depend heavily on contextual clues and on the redundancy of overused statements and directions in their early language comprehension. Adults learn to give many clues when communicating with young children, such as gestures, exaggerated stress, repetition and pointing as aids to comprehension, and children learn to utilize these clues (Bloom, 1974). This is not a significant problem except when attempting to measure specifically what part of the message the child understood linguistically. Even if the number of extralinguistic and suprasegmental clues is reduced it is still difficult to present language in a situation where the child must understand the structure of the sentence in order to respond correctly.

The evidence from some of the early comprehension studies, plus the difficulties in studying comprehension, have led to the assumption that comprehension precedes production every step of the way. It is, after all, difficult to think of understanding and speaking developing separately, with children possibly learning different rules for each. Bloom (1974), however, feels that while production of speech appears to depend on prior development of comprehension, it is not clear that the emergence of speech and understanding shadow each other. Most of the evidence about emerging comprehension in children comes from the early diary studies and is largely anecdotal.

Some of the recent studies, however, have produced evidence supporting Bloom's ideas. Lahey (as discussed by Bloom, 1974) investigated the use of prosody and syntactic markers in children's comprehension of spoken sentences. She compared 4- and 5-year-old children's comprehension of three complex structures; coordinated sentences, sentences with center-embedded relative clauses and right-branching relative clauses. It was found that coordinated sentences were easiest to understand and right-branching relative clauses the most difficult. Because the subjects included the syntactic marker while repeating and acting out the sentences, yet demonstrated no understanding of the sentence structure, Lahey concluded that children may incorporate surface features of the language into their speech before fully understanding the underlying meaning represented by the forms. Bloom (1974) concludes that there is presently not enough information available to explain the relationship between speaking and understanding language. The relationship between the two probably shifts and varies according to the experience of the child and his developing linguistic and cognitive capacities.

For the hearing-impaired child the important question is whether he can process the syntax of simple sentences, for instance, when he is not yet producing such syntactic structures. If there is such evidence for the child's comprehension of simple sentence structure, the basis exists for beginning work on the production of those sentences.

Even though the relationship may not be the simple comprehension-precedes-production that it was once thought to be, it is important that an assessment of comprehension in the hearing-impaired child is attempted. Some methods for assessing comprehension will be discussed later in the chapter. Before discussing evaluation tools, however, two special aspects of evaluation, usually conducted by necessity without the aid of formal evaluation instruments, should be briefly described. The first is the evaluation of the very young child in terms of his readiness for language acquisition.

ASSESSING READINESS FOR LANGUAGE ACQUISITION

The task of assessing a child's readiness for language development is a challenging one and there is little meaningful information or objective measures available to help in the process. Here, even more than in other assessment situations, one needs to be an acute observer of linguistic as well as nonlinguistic behavior. And, as mentioned earlier, although the concern is primarily with the child's readiness for language acquisition, it is extremely important to be sensitive to signs of other problems which may interfere with his acquisition of language.

Formal instruments are not usually applicable for the very young child and the evaluation is much more productive if conducted over a period of time and in varied situations. The most revealing observations will result from observing the child when he is at ease in a familiar situation with familiar people such as his parents and siblings. There is a tremendous amount of meaningful linguistic behavior that occurs before the child utters his first word and it is that behavior we want to assess.

Hearing-impaired children at ages 3 to 5 years will vary greatly in their behavior and their linguistic awareness. Such factors as the level of hearing loss, age at which the loss was discovered, age of hearing aid fitting and acceptance of aid, early education (parental guidance, auditory training) and, most importantly, the environment of the home will affect linguistic development.

Observation of General Behavior

One can begin evaluating the young child's development by observing some nonlinguistic indicators of developmental level. Is he aware of his surroundings and does he respond appropriately? What is the nature of his response to the environment and people? What kind of clues and stimuli does he attend to? Is it possible to establish eye contact with him and how long can he sustain attention? It is particularly revealing to observe what kind of communication has been established between the child, his parents and siblings.

One wants to generally observe what evidence there is of cognitive development in the child. There is a tremendous range in the quality of play activities, for instance, of a child at this age. Some children can engage in purposeful, organized play over a period of time. Another child's behavior might be random, disregarding the environment and without any obvious organization or purpose.

One observation of a 3-year-old child with developmental delay (according to psychological evaluation) and other handicaps besides deafness revealed that she was able to initiate and organize a "Tea party" situation and sustain this play for almost an hour. Obviously she will respond differently in the classroom than another 3-year-old child with whom it is impossible even to establish eye contact. It is important to consider the cognitive/linguistic relationship. Does the child attach a consistent linguistic representation in any mode to what he demonstrates that he understands about the world?

Another aspect of behavior to monitor is the establishment of a response set or habit. Has the child developed or is it possible to develop with him turn-taking behavior? In other words, will the child take part in simple games in which he must attend to the action of another person and respond with an appropriate action? The ability or inability of a child to engage in this kind of behavior is important in terms of how he will respond to classroom activities. This ability is an important precursor for attending to the language of others and for the turn-taking behavior (speaker/hearer relationship) that is basic to language development.

More specifically, it is important to observe the child's responsiveness to sound. Is he consistent in his response to those environmental sounds that are a regular and meaningful part of his environment? It should be noted here that this is an extremely difficult aspect of behavior to assess. Depending on the child's age and level of maturity and the length of time he has worn a hearing aid, his response to environmental sounds can vary widely from situation to situation. Attention plays a large part here, with factors such as fatigue and other distracting stimuli easily masking a child's response. One revealing bit of behavior often observed is that of the child, during play, imitating environmental sounds to accompany his play; for example, imitating the sound of a motor or machine as he pushes a toy car.

Observation of Linguistic Behavior

The most significant part of this assessment is observation of the child's linguistic awareness and communicative intent to determine whether the child has any understanding of the functions communication can serve and, more specifically, whether he realizes that communication is a two-way street. Does he expect to give and receive information via oral language, body language, gesture or manual communication? The mode in which the child communicates is not as important as whether or not he has an awareness of the purpose of language and the intent to communicate. And, if the child has this awareness and intention, how is it linguistically represented?

Long before any meaningful sounds or syllables are produced by the hearing infant, he produces a range of *noises* which signal his inner state. A young baby initially uses sound (cries and whimpers) not to communicate meaning but to signal his needs and physical states. Between the period of one to six weeks, undifferentiated crying becomes differentiated and, by six months, this vocalization has developed intonational form and purpose (Dale, 1976). Jakobson (1968) describes this development:

". . . . permanent speech sounds emerge from the babbling sounds, embryo-words emerge from the prelanguage residue. The persistence of the sound – the intention to express meaning by the formation in which it occurs and the social setting of the utterance are fundamental criteria for distinguishing speech sounds from babbling sounds" (p.29).

The next step in development is the jargon-like speech which is so intriguing because it seems the child is indeed communicating but in a language that we don't understand. This period, when the child reproduces the intonation patterns, rhythm and stress of the language he hears but with words that are for the most part unintelligible, is a very important part of language development. While the relationship between the development of segmental and suprasegmental aspects of language is not yet well understood, it is possible that suprasegmentals are the first to convey meaning (Dale, 1976). Simultaneously, a feeling for phrasing and sentence contours is established and the framework into which the structures of the language will be fitted begins to develop. While the acquisition of first words are probably more exciting to parents and easier for the professional to measure as a sign of progress, these suprasegmental aspects of language are perhaps more important in determining how far the child has progressed in laying the foundations for language acquisition.

Some of the questions to be answered are: Is the child producing sound and if so of what type and quality? That is, could his vocalizations be characterized as babbling with a range of sounds (consonants and vowels or approximations thereof) and some hint at intonation? This would obviously be a more advanced level of development than that of a child who is producing only undifferentiated involuntary sounds in response to inner feelings rather than as a response to the environment. And, what is the quality of the babbling? Does it resemble speech in its pitch and intensity, or is it flat, undifferentiated, and high pitched? Is the quality of the child's laugh and cry natural? Does he control the volume and pitch of his productions?

With the child who is producing strings of sound containing some contour, it is important to assess his contrastive use of intonation. Does he appropriately produce utterances of the following types?

(garble) ! (exclamation)

(garble) ? (interrogative)

(garble) . (declarative)

And, conversely, does he respond to the intonation patterns that he hears? Does he, for example, look around quizzically when the teacher says "Where is the ball?" Is he moved to action by "Go get the ball!"? Responses of this type are extremely encouraging because they offer some evidence that the child is developing a discrimination of sentence types by intonation pattern.

Another aspect of development to be assessed is the child's ability to imitate. Can he reproduce sounds, syllables, intonation patterns, rhythms or at least approximations of these units? Important to this task is the added ability of the child to distinguish when an imitation is expected and when another type of response is expected. It is not uncommon for children who have been exposed to modeling techniques to produce an imitation as an all-purpose linguistic response.

A final category to be considered is whether the child has developed a reliable correspondence between a meaning or referent and a representation of it at any level or in any mode: sound, syllable, word, approximation of a word, gesture or sign. Regardless of what unit he uses, does he reliably and consistently use that representation to refer to some object/person/action? That is, does he refer in a linguistic manner?

This, then, is the continuum used for assessing the hearing-impaired child's readiness for language acquisition. These are some of the prelinguistic features that can be noted as indices of the child's progress toward the beginning of language acquisition.

ASSESSMENT OF WRITTEN LANGUAGE

The second special aspect of assessment on the other end of the developmental continuum is the evaluation of written language. The developmental aspects of writing are discussed in Chapter 3, but it seems pertinent here to make a few points about the evaluation of writing skills.

When appropriate, written samples should be included as part of a language evaluation. It is important to know how well a student uses a language form serving different functions than those of oral expression. More and more is expected from students in the written mode as they progress through middle school and into high school, and it is important to identify those students who are having problems with the written mode of language.

The skill of reproducing one's oral language in written form has been generally seen as the last step in the acquisition of language skills. The hearing child comes to school having already attained almost complete mastery of his receptive and expressive oral language. To this basic language competence it is assumed he adds the skill of reading; that is, he learns to decode the written representation of oral language. Lastly, he learns to produce this written form himself, to encode. This view has been the traditional approach in teaching the acquired skills. However, in more recent years other ideas regarding the order of teaching writing (C. Chomsky, 1972) have been proposed and writing is now considered as more than simply the transcription of spoken language.

Writing is a complex skill or performance based on a combination of oral language and reading skills and on the necessary component of motor skills. Because of this complexity, care must be exercised in evaluating the written language of hearing-impaired children and in the importance placed on this aspect of language evaluation. It is tempting, at times, to place undue emphasis on evaluation of written language if the student's expressive language is relatively unintelligible.

An evaluation based on a student's written language alone, however, would be attending only to a very specialized part of his linguistic competence. Written language should always be considered in relation to the student's basic language competence; that is, how it relates to his other expressive modes. Based on the level of the student's oral or signed expressive language, the question is what can be reasonably expected from his or her written language.

The first problem is the method used to collect a writing sample. Depending on the age and language level of the student, the method of sampling may be the most difficult decision in a language evaluation. Many students who have not had much success with written language and find it to be a laborious process are reluctant to write in the artificial context of a test situation. When asked to respond to a picture stimulus, for instance, students may be intimidated or unmotivated. Presenting such a task to a student may result in a small and non-representative output. (*FIGURE 9.77*)

WRITTEN SAMPLES IN RESPONSE TO PICTURE/CLASS ASSIGNMENTS

The following is a comparison of written language produced by the same student in response to a picture stimulus in the testing situation (paragraph 1) and in response to a class assignment after reading and discussing A Farewell to Arms (paragraph 2).

PARAGRAPH 1.

A little boy was dreaming one night that he got up in the morning and ate breakfast. He got dress in his space uniform went in to his rocket, when he got on the moon, he made friends with the funny looking people.

PARAGRAPH 2.

Henry had to do what he did. If Henry didn't go to Switzerland he would have been arrested. So I think Henry thought he was right to go to Switzerland. I think his feelings were satisfied in a way because he escaped from the war and he had Catherine the one he loves with him. I think he is happy to be there cause he doesn't have to be arrested or go to war and also he can be with Catherine. I think he feels safe in Switzerland. He may think of his old friends but I don't think he would like to be any where else than Switzerland with Catherine.

FIGURE 9.77 Written samples in response to picture/class assignments.

A better approach is to collect language samples over a period of time, produced under varying conditions in response to a variety of tasks or assignments. A sample consisting of some letter writing, some diary-type material, and classroom assignments such as accounts of class activities or responses to literature gives a more balanced picture of the student's writing skills.

It is also important to consider how the task determines the output in evaluating writing samples. The length of a sample may be totally irrelevant since very often this is teacher determined. For instance, if the teacher hands out a piece of paper along with the assignment, students very often feel that their task is to write until they have filled the paper. One excellent way to gain perspective on a particular student's level of written language is to gather samples from the entire class as a basis for comparison. This kind of sample can be compared with standard written English as well as with the output of the other children in the group. Such data can also give some insight into how the class as a whole responded to a particular writing task.

There are several different levels to be considered when assessing written language. First one wants to look at the sentence level. Can the student express the underlying grammatical relationships in an order and with a system that conveys the message? Does he have a sense of what a sentence must contain? Where is he on the continuum of language acquisition? Perhaps he can produce good simple sentences but the syntax breaks down when he attempts complex structures. Or, perhaps he is using complex sentences but revealing some problems specific to the development of complexity. Problems with progression of tense, backward and forward pronominalization in adverbial clauses and relative clauses, referencing across sentence boundaries and the use of complementizers are some of the areas of difficulty at this level.

Some of the errors frequently encountered in written language are predictable, such as omission of grammatical morphemes and function words. Those elements that are so commonly omitted from spoken language will usually also be omitted from written language. What is needed is to determine how the omissions should be ranked in order of seriousness. For instance, if a student is writing syntactically well-structured simple sentences but displays surface structure problems with morphological endings, he has a less serious problem than the student whose simple sentences are unintelligible because of faulty word order. If it is not clear what a child is trying to express because of lack of word order, there is not much point in worrying about morphological endings or use of determiners. *(FIGURE 9.78)*

Samples of Written Language Illustrating Faulty Word Order

This level of language is not "correctable" in the usual sense because it is often not interpretable, even when the context is known.

Table is needle water.
Work the doctor.
Eye is the baby.
No, the mother the baby.
Table is mother.
Is you're the baby.
Mother love city father.
Table was the baby.
Happy the father was her.
Are needle the doctor.

FIGURE 9.78 Samples of written language illustrating faulty word order

On another level, if the student is producing connected discourse in his writing, what is the relationship between his sentences? Is he writing a list or does he have a sense of the structure of a paragraph? The following samples of students' writing illustrate problems at this level. (*FIGURE 9.79*)

For the student who reveals good sentence and paragraph structure in his writing,

Written Language Illustrating Progression Toward Paragraph Form

Unrelated sentences, written as a list.

Child #1. The pony is sad.
The children come in garage.
The girl's birthday today.
The dog run with the cat.
The mother hold umbrella.
The grandmother hold the cake.
The girl hold her doll.

List of sentences with some minimal relationship between sentences.

Child #2. The chairs fell.
The two boys are fighting.
The pony was sad.
The childrens didn't like the rain.
Many childrens are fool around.
The dishes are fell.
The candys fell.
The napkins fell.
The mother helps Grandmother cake.
Many childrens are all wet.

Child #3. The childrens came to house. Today is Alice's birthday. The childrens sat in the chair. When the rain came down, the childrens ran into the house. The stable got wet! The pony got wet! Hat got wet. The two boy are fighting.

Child #4. We had a birthday party in the garage, because it's rainy today. They think, "they should not ride a pony outside. The pony was sad. The children began to fool and fight because it's rainy. Two women came out of the door. There are five candles on the cake.

FIGURE 9.79 Samples of written language illustrating the progression toward a sense of paragraph form

the assessment then becomes a much more complex one. He is at a level where his writing can be evaluated in terms of story structure; that is, whether it contains a sense of narrative development and descriptive comment, and generally those aspects of writing go hand-in-hand with the developmental reading skills discussed in Chapter 4.

Evaluation Tools and Techniques

The preceding sections have discussed collecting data on the child's spontaneous use of language, some of the problems involved in this process and the importance of sampling the child's language in a variety of situations. This section discusses what can be learned through the use of formal tests, problems inherent in the testing situation and the advantages and disadvantages of specific tests.

While there are some definite limitations involved in any formal testing situation, particularly in attempting to elicit and sample language behavior in this way, there are also some advantages to interacting with the child in a structured, standardized situation. For one thing, standardized materials are good for comparing the performances of members of a group. While such a comparison may be invalid, as when comparing hearing-impaired children to hearing children, there are still occasions when standard scores become meaningful. Any time the same test or group of tests is administered to the members of a class, the teacher gains some valuable information for setting goals for the class as a whole or possibly for making changes in the group. Performance measured in a standardized situation offers the possibility of developing in-house norms which, among other things, could be used in evaluating the effectiveness of the curriculum being used.

The testing situation also makes it possible to observe how well the child can function linguistically with a minimum of extralinguistic clues. As discussed in the second section – collecting linguistic data – one aspect of language development is the progressive freeing of language comprehension from dependence on situational clues. An advantage of formal testing is it requires the child to use the pure linguistic data of the item rather than all the other clues available to him in a more natural situation.

Thus, the test situation provides information about two aspects of the child's linguistic functioning. One, it provides a baseline or a minimal assessment of the child's ability. If he can respond to an item (language structure) in the testing room, he probably, if motivated to do so, can respond in the classroom or living room. Two, the test situation provides some insight into how well the child has internalized the language presented to him and how well he can generalize that knowledge to new situations. For instance, if he has been exposed to relative clauses in the classroom and shows that he can correctly interpret this structure in the context of the familiar chart story, can he correctly interpret a relative clause when it is presented to him in a testing situation?

It is very important in the case of the hearing-impaired child to know if he can respond to and produce language that is not motivated by an immediate external event or by his internal state. Can he talk about other than the here-and-now and be understood by someone who is not familiar with the child's communication style? In other words, does the child have enough structure available to him to communicate a message to someone who doesn't already know the message?

There are some problems, however, inherent in the testing situation that should be considered at this point. The situation itself is so threatening for some children and so restrains their ability to respond that it is very difficult for them to produce any representative language or to respond according to their capability. It is very important to spend some time establishing a comfortable relationship with the child before testing begins. It is also good to begin with some nonthreatening tests, such as the ACLC (Assessment of Children's Language Comprehension) or the visual subtests of the ITPA (Illinois Test of Psycholinguistic Abilities) described in this section, that give the child an opportunity to develop confidence and achieve initial success. In spite of all possible preparation, however, some children are simply not able to function in a testing room. It is then necessary to do some creative thinking about how to make the situation more comfortable while still trying to get results.

Several solutions that have been used with some success are:

(1) To evaluate the child in a corner of his classroom or in some other room in which he is familiar and comfortable or to involve his teacher (or possibly his mother) in the testing procedure.

(2) To test two children together and record their interaction (which can be extremely revealing of communication style and level).

Yet it cannot be emphasized strongly enough that an assessment should never be based on the results of formal tests alone. Test results should always be considered in combination with data from the other situations described previously.

There are also specific aspects of formal tests that may be difficult for some children depending on their background and previous school experience. For instance, pictures are very often used in language tests and particularly in comprehension tests. Although this seems a reasonable task, children are not all equally able to respond to this kind of a format. Sigel, Anderson, and Shapiro (1966) found that lower-class black children had difficulty categorizing pictures of objects, while for middle-class black children the kind of representation (picture or object) made no difference. This can be a serious problem in testing children who are new to this culture and perhaps have had no previous school experience. It may be more valid, therefore, to test comprehension of sentence structure by using the picture format supplemented by some other method. One technique for testing comprehension is to use both the child's responses to pictures and his ability to manipulate objects in response to a stimulus sentence.

It is also important to analyze what is being required of the child by the test format

DIFFERENT TYPES OF RESPONSES TO ITPA GRAMMATIC CLOSURE SUBTEST

The following are examples of two different types of responses by students at the Rhode Island School for the Deaf to the Grammatic Closure subject of the ITPA. Child #1 demonstrates that he understands the task but cannot supply the correct morpheme, while Child #2 does not understand the task.

ITEM NO.	CHILD #1	CHILD #2
2 This cat is under the chair. Where is this cat? She is ______ .	top of the chair	sitting
4 This dog likes to bark. Here he is ______	bark	wool
6 The boy is opening the gate. Here the gate has been ______	open	school
8 This bicycle belongs to John. Whose bicycle is it? It is __________	John	bicycle
9 The boy is writing something. This is what he ______	writing	paper

Source: J. McCarthy & S. Kirk, *Illinois Test of Psycholinguistic Abilities*, Champaign: University of Illinois Press, 1961

FIGURE 9.80 Examples of two different types of responses to ITPA Grammatic Closure subtest

and what aspects of it may be either cognitively difficult or unnatural in the face of everyday language usage. For instance, in an experiment by Huttenlocher and Strauss (1968, as reported by Cazden, 1972), children were asked to create a pile of two blocks in response to the description, "The red block is on top of the green block," when one of the two blocks was in a fixed position and could not be manipulated. The task was much easier when the block that was free for the child to manipulate was the grammatical subject of the sentence (the red block). Evidently, when the green block (the object of the sentence) was the free one, children had to transform the statement to correspond to the extralinguistic situation before they could understand it.

The Grammatic Closure subtest of the ITPA is another example of a task that is very difficult for some children. This test requires the child to respond to pictures by "filling in the blank" with the necessary grammatical morpheme; for example, "Here is a bed. Here are two bed __ ." This completion task is very difficult for many hearing-impaired children as are most cloze-type tasks. They don't understand what is required of them as their sense of what constitutes a sentence is not formed well enough to allow them to determine what is missing. It is essential in such a situation to determine from the child's performance where the problem lies. If he responds with a grammatical morpheme but the incorrect one, the problem is less serious than if he cannot respond at all, or responds inappropriately with a word, for instance. *(FIGURE 9.80)*

Another problem often observed is that the more open-ended the task, the more difficult it will be for a hearing-impaired child. The child depends on both verbal and nonverbal context to narrow the possibility for response. Therefore, tasks which require him to respond to a picture with little direction and no context ("Tell me about this picture.") are not likely to result in a good representative sample of his language.

There are two important considerations when evaluating a child's behavior in the testing situation. First, the tasks required by the formal tests need to be analyzed in terms of what kinds of cognitive and linguistic challenges and problems they present. Second, the results must be considered in light of the fact that behavior in a testing room may be very different from behavior elsewhere. An estimation of the child's ability should be based on the total picture, never on performance of one kind of task.

On the ITPA Grammatic Closure subtest previously mentioned, the child's ability to supply the necessary morpheme does not guarantee that he uses these morphemes in his spontaneous language. And his use of a particular language form in a test situation may not mean that he understands the full range of its use. Even more importantly though, if a child is not able to supply the appropriate morpheme, one cannot assume that he never uses these morphemic structures. Perhaps in a more natural situation with a meaningful context, or when the most salient aspect of what he wants to express demands accurate morphology, he may indeed use these grammatical markers. If the results from this test, supplemented by results from comprehension testing and samples of his spontaneous written language, all indicate problems with grammatical morphemes, then there is solid evidence on which to base recommendations.

APPLICABILITY OF SPECIFIC TESTS

In spite of the limitations of standardized tests, there are some language tests and subtests that, when modified, can be very useful with hearing-impaired children. The point must be made again, however, that when there has been no test standardization using a hearing-impaired population, caution must be exercised when computing scores (age or grade equivalents) from test results.

The Assessment of Children's Language Comprehension Test (ACLC) (Foster, Giddan, & Stark, 1973) is a nonthreatening, easy-to-administer test which utilizes a picture format and requires only a pointing response. It incorporates the very desirable feature of first testing the vocabulary (50 items) to be used in testing progressively longer phrases. This test is very useful for young children whose comprehension might be limited and in establishing a baseline with a child who is being evaluated for the first time. However, it does not really test for sentence structure as the test items are phrases of up to four words (or critical elements) and it provides but a superficial estimate of language comprehension as all of the items pictured are concrete objects.

Another relatively comprehensive test utilizing a picture format is the Auditory Test for Language Comprehension (Carrow, 1968). The items on this test range from comprehension of isolated vocabulary items and morphological endings to comprehension of syntactical structures. It therefore tests a wide range of structures although it is a bit heavy on morphology and light on syntax. There are 101 items in all, some of which are very interesting since they are less concrete than the items usually found on tests utilizing the picture format.

For example, there are several items which provide a contrast by picturing a single object, two objects and many objects. On one item the stimulus word is a number, but on the others, stimulus words such as *some, many, a few,* or *pair* are used. There are a number of items which, because they test for discrimination of morphemes such as final *-s,* are particularly difficult for hearing-impaired subjects. Generally tests of this type are tests of lipreading for the profoundly hearing-impaired child and the attendant problems should be considered when evaluating the results.

Both the Carrow test and the ACLC have been used to test comprehension of signed English with children whose comprehension of oral language is extremely limited. It is often a useful technique to set up a comparative situation for evaluating the child's performance using oral language alone and then with the addition of sign. If it is helpful to know under what circumstances the child functions best, in what situation his comprehension is best, if he can function in an oral environment or needs the addition of sign, or to evaluate his comprehension generally when receiving input in two modes simultaneously, then a comparative situation yields helpful data. The only stipulation is to structure the situation carefully so the results will be clear. In other words, if one wants to evaluate comprehension of oral language, the input must be oral, not a combination of oral language, gestures and an approximation to signs.

It is feasible to utilize these tests using signed English although there are several ramifications of this procedure which should be considered:

(1) There are some items for which the signs are so iconic that it is really no longer a test of language comprehension.

(2) In regard to the saliency of the morphological endings, there is a tremendous difference between presenting the items orally and presenting them with the addition of sign. While the final *-s* is very difficult to lipread, it is almost overemphasized when signed. It is important in this situation to determine whether the child, who understands plurality when it is signed to him, can ever detect plurality in an oral situation with the help of contextual clues.

(3) If you wish to evaluate the child's comprehension of language structure, then the question of mode really is a secondary one. The basic question is whether the child understands language structure and secondly, what kind of input (oral and/or signed) is necessary for comprehension.

The Carrow test can also be administered in Spanish and has been administered in Portuguese. In fact, some interesting contrastive data have emerged from this testing. For example, it is easier for hearing-impaired children to distinguish the plural morpheme /s/ in Portuguese than in English since /s/ in final position in Portuguese becomes /sh/ and therefore easier to lipread, probably because it is rounded.

The Peabody Picture Vocabulary Test (PPVT) (Dunn, 1965) is also a test of receptive vocabulary utilizing a picture format and, therefore, a test of lipreading ability as well. The limitation of this test for use with hearing-impaired children is that the vocabulary quickly becomes too difficult and the test reveals nothing about the child's comprehension of language structure. Also, the PPVT is often used as a general intelligence test since its scores correlate highly with the Stanford-Binet intelligence scores, but would result in an extremely unreliable estimation of a hearing-impaired child's intelligence since vocabulary would not be a reasonable index of his overall intellectual ability.

One of the most commonly used language tests is the Illinois Test of Psycholinguistic Abilities (Paraskevopoulos and Kirk, 1969). It is based on a theory of three dimensions of language behavior: modality, type of process and level of organization (Osgood, 1957). In spite of its popularity, some of the test's subtests have little to do with language (the Visual Closure test or Manual Expression, for instance) and none of the subtests assess comprehension or production of syntactic structures. Subtests such as Auditory Closure and Sound Blending are obviously not appropriate for use with hearing-impaired children, and while others, such as the Auditory Memory test, can be adminstered to these children, the normative data included would not be very relevant.

Some of the visual subtests, however, provide an interesting format for determining how the child is functioning cognitively. In

ORAL/WRITTEN RESPONSES TO ITPA GRAMMATIC CLOSURE SUBTEST

ITEM NO.	CORRECT RESPONSE	ORAL RESPONSE	WRITTEN RESPONSE
1	dogs	dog	dogs
5	dresses	dress	dresses
8	John's	John	John's
16	biggest	big	biggest
30	leaves	leave	leaves
31	children	children	childreds*
33	themselves	themselves	themselfs*

*This procedure also sometimes reveals uncertainty about spelling words that are used correctly orally.

FIGURE 9.81 Examples of oral and written responses from the same student to the Grammatic Closure subtest of the ITPA

these cases it would be useful to know how the child compares to a hearing child of a comparable age. The Visual Reception and Visual Association tests, for instance, are usually fun for the child and certainly are not intimidating. They provide a good starting place for the examiner who is unfamiliar with the child being tested. The tests require no verbal response and have been used successfully with very young children and with children who have very limited expressive language. The one limitation, however, is they are not appropriate for use with children who are new to the culture as the items seem to be culturally bound. The Visual Sequential Memory subtest also provides some idea of how the child is functioning visually.

The ITPA Grammatic Closure subtest mentioned before is a test that uses a completion task to elicit grammatical morphemes. This does not work well with young children, as they have difficulty understanding the requirements of the task. But, used with older children, particularly late middle school and early high school age, this test may be helpful in deciding how well they are acquiring the less salient (difficult to perceive auditorily and to lipread) aspects of language. However, it is sometimes difficult to determine if children are actually articulating some of the morphemes (such as final -s). To overcome this problem, the child may be asked to respond in writing as well as orally. By adapting the test this way one gains some perspective on the relationship between the child's expressive language in two different modes. Often a child who does not articulate morphemes in final position (to make them understandable to the listener) is indeed aware of these aspects of language and will produce them in written language.

One other technique which can be used to sample language is imitation. A considerable amount of research has been done using both spontaneous imitation and elicited imitation to acquire data on the child's use of structures that may rarely appear in his spontaneous language. Dale (1976) gives a good account of some of this research and the uses of this technique.

It is important to keep in mind the difference between spontaneous and elicited imitation and what the implications are for using this technique in a testing situation. In discussing spontaneous imitation, Dale (1976) concludes that the evidence of Bloom, Hood, and Lightbown (1974), and of Kemp and Dale (1973), demonstrate that:

"imitation is a selective process that represents the 'growing edge' of language. It may serve a useful function in firmly establishing new aspects of language, but it is not the means by which the child picks up new features" (p. 117).

The important point is, if in elicited as well as spontaneous imitation the child can produce only what he can produce in his spontaneous language (as is commonly believed), this technique can be used to gather further data regarding the child's production and comprehension of language.

The advantage of using elicited imitation as a tool for evaluation is that one can test specific structures and also progressively longer and more complex structures to determine just how much a child can process. The underlying rationale is that children will process sentences that exceed auditory memory span according to how much they know about language structure. One can, therefore, tell how much the child understood of such sentences by looking at how much is preserved in his repetition; if a sentence is too long to hold in short-term memory (and therefore cannot be easily repeated), he will process the meaning and perhaps restructure it in his production. The results reflect evidence of how much the child understood and what he knows about reproducing the meaning. It is, in a sense, a way of sampling both comprehension and production with one technique.

The Elicited Language Inventory Test (Carrow, 1974) is widely used to study imitation. While it is appropriate for use with older hearing-impaired children, it includes too few short, syntactically simple sentences for use with younger children.

Imitation testing is one situation in which the teacher can design her own test sentences using vocabulary with which the child is familiar, so his ability to reproduce the structure of the sentence can be assessed. Unfamiliar vocabulary is therefore eliminated and does not interfere with the child's reproduction of the structure. The length and complexity of sentences should stretch the child's memory somewhat. If the sentence does not exceed the child's auditory memory span, responses may be merely echoed and reveal nothing about his understanding of the sentence. He will be able to perform the task without processing the meaning of the sentence. A series of sentences which increase gradually in length and in complexity but retain familiar vocabulary will provide a means of determining precisely where performance begins to break down. *(FIGURE 9.82)*

Slobin and Welsh (1973) used elicited imitation as a research tool and their article is well worth reading as background informa-

SENTENCES INDICATING INCREASING LENGTH/COMPLEXITY

Simple sentences of increasing length

John fell.
The dog runs.
The baby is crying.
The girl hit the boy.
The boy threw the ball.
The boy is eating the apple.
Bill gave an apple to the teacher.
Bill opened the door with a key.
The boy threw the ball over the car.
The children are picking apples from the tree.

Complex sentences of increasing length

Bill is small but strong.
It was Bill Mary hit.
The car Father bought was old.
What John did was hit Bill.
The cat the dog chased was black.
The girl hit the boy and ran away.
The boy hit the girl and she cried.
Because he was dirty Bill took a bath.
While the children ate lunch, mother washed the dishes.
The teacher gave books to the children who were sitting down.

FIGURE 9.82 *Sentences indicating increasing length of sentence and increasing complexity*

tion for constructing an imitation task. They caution that what is missing in this type of linguistic task are intention and context. This should be kept in mind when evaluating the child's performance. In the absence of these factors, the imitation task can strain the child's abilities and therefore his performance must be considered as only a conservative estimate of his linguistic competence.

The point being made about all of these tests is that they furnish a method and the materials with which to examine some specific aspects of language development. For the purpose of evaluating the linguistic development of hearing-impaired children though, the task must be carefully examined and the appropriateness of its use evaluated. It should be determined how the task differs in this situation from its use with hearing children and, finally, whether or not it is fair to compare the child's performance with those of hearing children by using the norms provided with the test. In most cases it is not meaningful to compute scores or profiles and it is usually not necessary. The performance of the child can be described as well as his response to these particular test materials, and that information can be added to all the other kinds of data collected to achieve a composite picture of the child's linguistic functioning. Numerical scores are rarely as meaningful as a narrative account for describing how the child functions in response to the materials and the task.

This discussion of testing materials is not meant to provide a list of specific tests which should be administered to every child evaluated. Rather, the evaluation process should be a creative one in which the child and the situation is assessed to determine what kind of information would be relevant and helpful. The first step should always be to review the existing information, consider the total picture and then choose those testing materials and techniques which will provide the most relevant data.

EVALUATION OF DATA

This section discusses ways of evaluating the data collected from sampling spontaneous language production and language comprehension.

Various methods can be used to quantify or reduce data to numbers in order to compare individual children and groups of children. One such method is the mean length of utterance (MLU) referred to in Chapter 2 and described by Brown (1973). Many questions have been raised about the validity, reliability and informativeness of this measure when applied to the language of normal children. These questions are discussed in detail by Cazden (1972) and several of these will be considered in this section.

Any quantification method that utilizes length as the unit to be measured counts units as if they were all alike and as if they carried the same weight in the sentence. This is not true, however, of words or morphemes because of the internal structure of the sentence. For example, one cannot compare the child's ability to sequence numbers or abstract visual configurations with his ability to sequence linguistic units in a sentence. Knowing that the child can repeat four digits or order a string of four abstract symbols (on the ITPA subtests) reveals something about the function of his auditory and visual memory. However, it may not tell us anything about how his memory for linguistic units functions. There is no way to compare the two performances because the sentence contains internal structure while a sequence of numbers or visual patterns does not.

Also, the morphemes in a sentence have different cognitive and semantic weight depending on the structural complexity of the sentence. And it is this structural complexity one wants reflected in any measure used to describe and evaluate a child's language. The MLU also fails to reveal anything about the function of a child's language – what he can or cannot do with his language.

The MLU presents other problems too when used to measure the development of a hearing-impaired child's language. The picture presented would be a misleading one masking the fact that, as the mean length of utterance increases, there are essential elements not being expressed. There would be no meaningful comparison between a hearing-impaired child's MLU and a hearing child's MLU because the former would consist primarily of content words and include very few of the grammatical morphemes which are such an important part of development in the early stages.

Cazden (1972) touches on this in her discussion of problems encountered when studying a group's language that differs markedly from standard English. Measuring development against such a standard interferes with recognizing the progress of this group.

Another problem in attempting to apply quantitative measures to linguistic data is that utilizing measures, such as the number of transformations to determine degree of complexity, does not have any solid experimental evidence to support it. The attempt to measure syntactic complexity cannot be separated from and may not parallel psychological complexity and cognitive processing of sentences (Fodor & Garrett, 1967; Bever, 1970). There is no reason to believe that all transformations carry equal psychological or cognitive/semantic weight. Therefore, efforts to describe a child's use of complex structures in terms of number of transformations may seriously distort or mask the relevant aspects of his use of those structures. This is particularly true with the developing language of the hearing-impaired child since we do not know what cognitive gaps he may have that will be reflected in his language development.

For example, transformations such as negation and question formation would seem to carry enormous cognitive/semantic weight since they are almost always expressed by very young hearing-impaired children. The form used to express these meanings, though, is usually less than fully developed. Transformations such as the passive, on the other hand, do not develop spontaneously in the language of hearing-impaired children and many exposures to this structure are necessary for acquisition (see Chapter 5). If the language description is to be useful and productive it should be based on what is typical of the language development for that particular group (in this case, the hearing impaired) and should reflect how we can utilize their language base to further develop a complete language system.

Measuring only deviance from the norms of a developmental sequence of language for the hearing child is not a suitable guide. The criterion should be the linguistic system that is to be acquired, not a comparison with the development of some other group. The problems in describing or analyzing the language of profoundly hearing-impaired children are so pervasive and so tied to the cognitive/semantic aspects of language development that none of the schemes used to measure development in hearing children are really appropriate. In addition, many of the texts which deal with language assessment utilize such rigidly structured approaches and complicated inventories that assessment becomes an overwhelming task for the teacher. This chapter is meant to be a guide to language assessment rather than a system or inventory.

Crystal et al. (1976) criticizes the Lee and Canter scoring technique (1971), for example, as too inflexible since it does not allow for varying degrees of grammatical completeness – a structure is not scored unless all of the required syntactic and morphological rules have been observed – and thus precludes what can be learned from a child's errors. A consistent error can tell us much about the syntactical rules the child is using.

Language inventories also rarely allow for recording the context of the utterance. In the case of hearing-impaired subjects, context is usually necessary not only to interpret the meaning of the utterance but also to determine how the child functions with his language. Crystal is also critical of researchers who list syntactic features in a language assessment but do not relate them to any framework or grammatical model. This practice results in a tendency to describe those features which are easiest to describe (such as morphology) with no rationale for the selection of those particular features.

The concern should be with more fundamental problems than whether the child is expressing determiners appropriately or using correct subject-verb agreement. As Crystal et al. (1976) point out, the use of syntax scores are usually of little diagnostic value and the scoring system sometimes takes over when one is forced to fit every utterance into the scheme of such a system. Language inventories by themselves provide no explanation, no sense of system and, more importantly, no hierarchy against which one can measure the linguistic progress of a student.

As stated earlier, the approach taken here is to place the child on the developmental continuum described in Chapters 2 through 6. This approach to language development is based on a Chomsky-type transformational grammar and utilizes stages (or levels) to describe language acquisition. It is hoped that using these broader categories will help to avoid focusing solely on the less profound aspects of language such as subject-verb agreement, use of articles, adverbs and surface structure morphology. All of these problems have to be attended to eventually, but initial concern must be placed on the more basic aspects of language such as use of word order to express basic grammatical relations.

A first step in evaluating the data acquired, therefore, is to determine where the child is functioning receptively and expressively on the continuum: prelinguistic stage (as described earlier), single word stage, simple sentence stage, or complex sentence stage. A second step is to evaluate his language within one of these stages according to a hierarchy (or scale) of the aspects of language to be acquired ranked according to their importance in the system. In other words, just as all transformations don't carry the same cognitive/semantic weight, all the morphemes in a sentence cannot be weighed equally. This is also true when attempting to evaluate and put into perspective all aspects of the total linguistic functioning of the child.

To arrive at a hierarchy one can first identify a set of basic aspects of language essential to linguistic development. Categories such as the following can be grouped according to the stage at which they operate:

A. Simple sentence level:

1. Use of word order to express basic meanings such as subject-verb, subject-verb-object, subject-verb-indirect object, object.
2. Development of sentence modalities; declarative, interrogative, negative and imperative.
3. Development of time concepts as evidenced in verb phrase and adverbials.
4. Development of space concepts as evidenced in locative prepositional phrases.
5. Development of concept of attribute (use of adjectives).
6. Ability to reference (pronominalization).
7. Development of concept of number (in verb phrase and plural morpheme) and possession.

B. Complex sentence level:

1. Coordination (beginning with phrases and developing into ordering and sequencing of events by coordination of sentences).
2. Complex conceptions of space and time as evidenced in adverbial clauses.
3. Development of causal, relational and conditional concepts as evidenced in adverbial clauses.
4. More complex expression of attribute (use of relative clauses).

LANGUAGE RESPONSES TO PICTURE TESTS

PICTURE	CHILD'S RESPONSE	INTERPRETATION (from knowledge of context)
rabbit	home	I have a rabbit at home.
duck	duck	naming
boy scout	camp	I went to camp.
dog	dog	naming
baby	cute	The baby is cute.
cake	party	We had a party.
cake	eat	I ate cake.
classmate	sick	Mary is sick.
water	swim	I went swimming.
house	house	naming
airplane	airplane	naming

FIGURE 9.83 Language samples in response to pictures illustrating the contrast between naming and one word ideas.

5. Embedding of one sentence in another (relative clauses and noun phrase complementation).
6. Complex referencing (backward and forward pronominalization in complex sentences).
7. Deletion of redundant elements (in coordinated sentences, for example).

The foregoing list is not meant to be an exhaustive set of categories, but rather to illustrate the type and level of category to be considered. For example, at this step in the evaluation of data one might be concerned with the child's development of expression of time as revealed by his use of the verb phrase but would not necessarily focus on the particular form used. It would be important to note whether he was making a conceptual distinction between present action and past action or present action and progressive action without being overly concerned with the form the expression takes. One may identify which of these fundamental aspects of language the child is expressing exclusive of what mode he is using for expression or what kind of structure, if any, he is using.

The next step is to describe what particular structure (in linguistic terms) the child is using to express these basic concepts and the difference between his structure and the standard desired. A final step of the evaluation is to outline the steps needed to narrow the gap between his linguistic representation and the standard linguistic representation.

Some examples might be useful to illustrate these points. For instance, if it is found that a child is functioning at a one-word stage there are many aspects of language that are not relevant to this particular evaluation, but it is important to know how he uses his one word. Is he **naming** (a very basic aspect of the use of one word)? Or is he expressing a one-word idea by using the word plus context and extra-linguistic features such as suprasegmentals and body language? *(FIGURE 9.83)* Is the child using suprasegmental marking or an intonation contour with his word? Does he use contrastive marking which would allow some interpretation? How many of the sentence modalities described above could be attributed to him on the basis of his intonation? That is, is it possible to distinguish between his use of a word to express an interrogative versus an imperative sentence type? Is the child producing his word for communication purposes? Does he have an intent to communicate or does he mostly imitate? Observations of this kind can help to describe what his one-word expression reveals about his cognitive level. And what about comprehension? Does he show that he understands utterances of greater length and complexity than one word?

It is indeed difficult to interpret and analyze the purpose and meaning of the child's one-word expression. More research needs to be done with hearing children to determine what concepts they have mastered and are expressing at this stage. However, with careful use of contextual and situational information, it should be possible to extract meaningful data about the child's use of one-word utterances.

Other examples can be drawn from the simple sentence stage. There are many aspects of language to be considered at this level, which is a crucial stage of development for the child since his subsequent progress will be based on this simple sentence stage. When considering a child who uses four-to five-word utterances, many of the concepts suggested in the previous outline A (simple sentence level), should be apparent in his language.

The following are some of the questions to be asked at this level:

(1) How many of the simple sentence patterns described in Chapter 4 are reliably expressed? The first consideration is to examine the word order of the utterances, since this is basic to the ability to signal unambiguously the relationships in a simple sentence. If the child is using an atypical word order, then it should be determined if he has a system at all or is using more or less random order.

It is important not only to consider if the child is producing a pattern three sentence for example, but in a more basic sense if he expresses attribute. What should be noted is not just the use of the sentence patterns per se, but what it reveals about the child's conceptual development.

(2) How many of the basic sentence modalities does the child express (i.e., declarative, negative, interrogative, imperative)? It is likely that most of these sentence types are being attempted, as well as perhaps some simple coordination of phrases. But it is unlikely that any type of recursion or embedding would be expressed.

(3) What particular form is being used to express the sentence types? For example, if question forms are expressed, do they include appropriate use of do-support? Does this extend to use of do-support in negation, or does the negative consist of an all-purpose "not"?

(4) After studying the particular ways in which the child expresses basic concepts, one might consider morphology in general, knowing that certain aspects of morphology are predictably difficult for a hearing-impaired child to acquire and use consistently. For instance, the final-*s* (table*s*, girl'*s*, goe*s*) is very often not expressed, but most consistently is missing from the third-person singular verb form *goes* because, in this case, it carries very little semantic weight.

The important point is not that these morphemes are so predictably missing in the hearing-impaired child's language, but to determine the significance of these omissions. If a child demonstrates comprehension of plurality and possessiveness but does not signal it linguistically, this problem is less serious than if he does not understand plurality. Similarly, if a child does not express the past tense *-ed*, does it mean that he does not have past tense markers in his expressive language? Or, does it reflect a cognitive problem with time? It is a superficial problem if it is merely an inability to mark tense overtly, but profound if it reflects a cognitive problem.

At this point, omission of function words could be considered. An example of a difficult cognitive structure to acquire is the definite indefinite determiner. To acquire an intuition for the use of determiners without being exposed to the many examples on which a hearing child bases his acquisition is exceedingly difficult. This is corroborated by the difficulty Japanese adults experience in learning English. The Japanese language does not utilize the definite/indefinite distinction and it is very difficult to acquire this concept as an adult language learner.

These examples are to emphasize that in every case, one must look not only at the child's surface structure (what he overtly expresses) but also at the set of rules the child is operating with and how they reflect his cognitive development. Knowing that hearing-impaired children almost always manifest morphological problems should not mean that one concentrates exclusively on this aspect of linguistic functioning. Rather, one must determine what level of functioning such morphological problems reflect in regard to their importance in the acquisition of language as a whole.

At the complex sentence level all of these points should be considered, plus the problems which are peculiar to the development of complexity. There are other aspects of language which become important to evaluate in addition to the development of complex linguistic structures. The cognitive and semantic considerations discussed in Chapter 6 are crucial to the development of complex structures and are discussed in depth in that chapter. It is more important than ever to consider not just surface structure problems, but what they reveal about the cognitive growth of the child and his ability to organize the world. Event ordering rather than simple sequencing and the ability to express relationships between attributes and events are examples of the level of concept to be evaluated.

The sample language evaluation which follows illustrates how the approach to evaluation and the tests and techniques utilized are chosen to fit the particular child and situation. *(FIGURE 9.84)*

ACKNOWLEDGMENTS

Many of the ideas in this chapter were first outlined in the appendix to *Child Language and Eduation* by Courtney B. Cazden. The authors also wish to thank Professor Cazden for her other contributions to the Rhode Island School for the Deaf Language Curriculum. Comments and criticism about this chapter by Professor Sheila Blumstein, Brown University, are appreciated by the authors.

LANGUAGE EVALUATION

CLASS OBSERVATION

L is smaller and younger than the other students in the class. He also is the only boy in this group. He seems, however, to be functioning well, is much more attentive than in his previous placement and does not seem bothered by these differences.

Linguistically *L* seems to have two quite different communication styles in the classroom. In a structured classroom situation he can produce very intelligible or well-constructed simple sentences and some complex sentences. Although he has trouble sequencing longer, more complex structures, he can usually correct his errors with a little help and encouragement. He was observed to produce complex sentences containing adverbial clauses and infinitives in this situation.

In communication with other students *L* uses much more telegraphic language with very little structure.

Receptively *L* functions much better in a structured situation than in unstructured, open-ended conversation. His comprehension of questions in particular is poor unless he has a framework and some expectations about what is being questioned.

He was also noted to be having problems with pronoun shift. For example, if the teacher says "I like your shirt," *L* is uncertain whether he should model that sentence or shift perspective to "I like my shirt."

TEST RESULTS

Assessment of Children's Language Comprehension. *L* performed well on this test, as might be expected since the stimulus range is from isolated vocabulary words up to four-word phrases. He scored 100% correct on the vocabulary and two-word phrases, 90% on three-word phrases and 60% on four-word phrases. Although he did not do well on longer phrases this can at least partly be attributed to his impulsivity.

Carrow Comprehension Test. In this test *L* responded poorly to those items that required interpretation of morphological endings, complex verb phrases and syntactic structure. Although some of these responses are predictable, such as his response to plural *s*, the test also revealed that he cannot interpret the information carried by past tense and past perfect endings or the structure of passive and dative sentences. Again, his impulsivity interfered with his performance.

The test was administered again several weeks later with the addition of sign. Although *L* responded correctly to many more of the single vocabulary items, he did as poorly as before with morphological endings, complex verb phrases and passive and dative structures. It was clearly not a case of *L* missing these items because of difficulty with comprehension of oral language, but rather because he does not understand the structure.

Carrow Imitation Test. This test requires imitation of sentences ranging from simple two-word sentences to eight-word complex sentences. *L*'s response was consistent with his response in other areas in that he was best able to reproduce a simple subject-verb-object structure. With longer and more complex sentences he shortens and sometimes simplifies (by omitting function words) and often changes the meaning. As an example, he repeats a passive sentence in the active form, and changes datives to a simple SVO structure.

Language Board. *L* was asked to read sentences and illustrate them by manipulating objects and figures. His performance was again consistent. He was able to illustrate simple sentences, but not passives or complex sentences containing relative clauses.

On a test of reading comprehension *L*'s performance was erratic because his problem with comprehension of question forms interfered with the task. He was able to answer correctly the simplest who, what and where informational questions, but he could not answer a verbal question (What did he do?) or a yes/no question and he persisted in giving noun phrase answers. It seems more likely, therefore, that he didn't understand the question than that he didn't understand what he read.

WRITTEN LANGUAGE

L is able to write well-structured simple sentences, although he does not always do so. His performance seems to depend on the assignment, which is also true of the other students in the class. They too sometimes produce faulty sentences with garbled word order and omissions of various types.

L is attempting complex sentences in his most recent written work but not successfully. His written language is lagging behind his oral ability, which is not surprising as he does not have the tools for sentence combining. This is reflected by his problems with word order in complex sentences.

SUMMARY

The test results show consistently that *L* functions well on a simple sentence level. At this stage in his development he is attempting to use complex sentences and is more successful orally than in his written language. He is also much more successful in a structured situation than in spontaneous casual conversation.

RECOMMENDATIONS

1. Continued work on comprehension of question forms. *L* is very uncertain in this area and this will impede his progress greatly as more is demanded of him at higher levels.
2. Structured language work to help *L* develop complex sentences. He has demonstrated the use of adverbial clauses and infinitives but he needs work on other types of complex sentences such as passive, relative clauses, noun phrase complements, pronominalization, dative, the various types of conjunction.
3. Continued work on written language to help *L* incorporate the structures he can use orally into his written language.

BIBLIOGRAPHY

Baird, R. On the role of chance in imitation-comprehension-production test results. *Journal of Verbal Learning and Verbal Behavior,* 1972, *11,* 474–477.

Bar-Adon, A., & Leopold, W. (Eds.). *Child language: A book of readings.* Englewood Cliffs, NJ: Prentice Hall, 1971.

Bellugi, U., & Klima, E. S. Aspects of sign language and its structure. In J. Kavanaugh & J. E. Cutting (Eds.), *The role of speech in language.* Cambridge, MA: M.I.T. Press, 1975.

Berko, J. The child's learning of English morphology. *Word,* 1958, *14,* 150–177.

Bever, T. G. The cognitive basis for linguistic structures. In J. R. Hayes (Ed.), *Cognition and the development of language.* New York: Wiley, 1970.

Blackwell, P., & Engen, E. Language curriculum for handicapped learners. In F. Withrow & C. Nygren (Eds.), *Language materials and curriculum management for the handicapped learner.* Columbus, OH: Merrill Publishing, 1976.

Blackwell, P., & Hamel, C. *The language curriculum: Rhode Island School for the Deaf,* 1971.

Bloom, L. M. A comment on Lee's "Developmental sentence types: A method for comparing normal and deviant syntactic development." *Journal of Speech and Hearing,* 1967, *32,* 294–296.

Bloom, L. M. *Language development: Form and function in emerging grammars.* Cambridge, MA: M.I.T. Press, 1970.

Bloom, L. M. *One word at a time: The use of single word utterances before syntax.* The Hague: Mouton, 1973.

Bloom, L. M. Talking, understanding and thinking. In R. L. Schiefelbusch & L. L. Lloyd (Eds.), *Language perspectives: Acquisition, retardation and intervention.* Baltimore: University Park Press, 1974.

Bloom, L. M., Hood, L., & Lightbown, P. Imitation in language development: When and why. *Cognitive Psychology,* 1974, *6,* 380–420.

Bond, G., & Wagner, E. *Teaching the child to read.* New York: McMillan Co., 1966.

Bormuth, J. R. Readability: A new approach. *Reading Research Quarterly,* 1966, *1,* 79–132.

Bormuth, J. R., Manning, J., Carr, J., & Pearson, D. Children's comprehension of between- and within-sentence syntactic structures. *Journal of Educational Psychology,* 1970, *61,* 349–357.

Bowerman, M. *Early syntactic development: A cross-linguistic study with special reference to Finnish.* Cambridge, MA: Cambridge University Press, 1973.

Braine, M.D.S. The ontogeny of English phrase structure: The first phase. *Language,* 1963, *39,* 1–13.

Braine, M. D. S. On learning the grammatical order of words (1967). In L. Jacobovits & M. Miron (Eds.), *Readings in the psychology of language.* Englewood Cliffs, NJ: Prentice Hall, 1969.

Braine, M.D.S. On two types of models of the internalization of grammars. In D. Slobin (Ed.), *The ontogenesis of grammar: A theoretical symposium.* New York: Academic Press, 1971.

Brewer, W. F. Is reading a letter-by-letter process? In J. Kavanaugh & I. Mattingly (Eds.), *Language by ear and by eye.* Cambridge, MA: M.I.T. Press, 1972.

Bronowski, J., & Bellugi, U. Language, name and concept. *Science,* 1970, *168,* 669–673.

Brown, R. The development of wh-questions in child speech. *Journal of Verbal Learning and Verbal Behavior,* 1968, *7,* 279–290.

Brown, R. *A first language: The early stages.* Cambridge, MA: Harvard University Press, 1973.

Brown, R., Cazden, C., & Bellugi, U. The child's grammar from I to III. In J. P. Hill (Ed.), *1967 Minnesota Symposium on Child Psychology.* Minneapolis: University of Minnesota Press, 1969.

Brown, R., Fraser, C., & Bellugi, U. Explorations in grammar evaluation. In U. Bellugi & R. Brown (Eds.), *The acquisition of language. Monographs of the Society for Research in Child Development,* 1964, *29,* 79–92.

Brown, R., & Hanlon, C. Derivational complexity and order of acquisition in child speech. In J. R. Hayes (Ed.), *Cognition and the development of language.* New York: Wiley & Sons, 1970.

Bruner, J. S. *The process of education.* Cambridge, MA: Harvard University Press, 1960.

Bruner, J. S. *Toward a theory of instruction.* Cambridge, MA: Harvard University Press, 1966.

Bruner, J. S. *Beyond the information given.* New York: Norton & Co., 1973.

Bruner, J. S. The ontogenesis of speech acts. *Journal of Child Language,* 1975, *2,* 1–25.

Bruner, J. S., Goodnow, J., & Austin, G. *A study of thinking.* New York: Science Editions, Inc., 1967.

Bruner, J. S., Oliver, R., & Greenfield, P. *Studies in cognitive growth.* New York: Wiley & Sons, 1966.

Caniglia, J., Cole, N., Howard, W., Krohn, E., & Rice, M. *Apple tree: A developmental language program.* Beaverton, OR: Dormac, Inc., 1973.

Carroll, J. B., & Freedle, R. O. *Language comprehension and the acquisition of knowledge.* New York: Wiley & Sons, 1972.

Carrow, M. W. The development of auditory comprehension of language structure in children. *Journal of Speech and Hearing Disorders,* 1968, *33,* 99–111.

Cazden, C. B. *Environmental assistance to the child's acquisition of grammar.* Unpublished doctoral dissertation, Harvard University, 1965.

Cazden, C. B. The acquisition of noun and verb inflections. *Child Development,* 1968, *39,* 433–448.

Cazden, C. B. *Child language in education.* New York: Holt, Rinehart & Winston, 1972.

Cazden, C. B. Play with language and metalinguistic awareness: One dimension of language experience. In C. Winsor (Ed.), *Dimensions of language experience.* New York: Agathon Press, 1975.

Chafe, W. *Meaning and the structure of language.* Chicago: University of Chicago Press, 1970.

Chall, J. *Learning to read: The great debate.* New York: McGraw-Hill, 1967.

Chapman, R. S., & Miller, J. F. Word order in early two- and three-word utterances: Does production precede comprehension? *Journal of Speech and Hearing Research,* 1975, *18,* 355–371.

Chomsky, C. Write now, read later. In C. B. Cazden (Ed.), *Language in early childhood education.* Washington, DC: Nat'l Assoc. for the Educ. of Young Children, 1972.

Chomsky, N. *Syntactic structures.* The Hague: Mouton, 1957.

Chomsky, N. *Aspects of the theory of syntax.* Cambridge, MA: M.I.T. Press, 1965.

Chomsky, N. A review of B. F. Skinner's *Verbal Behavior* (1964). In J. Fodor & J. Katz (Eds.), *The structure of language: Readings in the philosophy of language.* Englewood Cliffs, NJ: Prentice-Hall, 1965.

Chomsky, N. *Cartesian linguistics.* New York: Harper & Row, 1966.

Chomsky, N. *Language and mind.* New York: Harcourt, Brace, Jovanovich, 1968.

Chomsky, N. *Topics in the theory of generative grammar.* The Hague: Mouton, 1969.

Clark, E. V. What's in a word? On the child's acquisition of semantics in his first language. In T. E. Moore (Ed.), *Cognitive development and the acquisition of language.* New York: Academic Press, 1973.

Clark, H. Space, time, semantics and the child. In T. E. Moore (Ed.), *Cognitive development and the acquisition of language.* New York: Academic Press, 1973.

Crystal, D., Fletcher, P., & Garman, M. *The grammatical analysis of language disability: A procedure for assessment and remediation.* New York: Elsevier Press, 1976.

Dale, P. S. *Language development: Form and function.* New York: Holt, Rinehart & Winston, 1976.

Darwin, C. Biographical sketch of an infant (1877). In A. Bar-Adon and W. Leopold (Eds.), *Child language: A book of readings.* Englewood Cliffs, NJ: Prentice Hall, 1971.

Davis, F. B. Research in comprehension in reading. *Reading Research Quarterly,* 1968, *3,* 499–545.

Dunn, L. *Peabody picture vocabulary test.* Minneapolis: American Guidance Service, 1965.

Egoff, S., Stubbs, G., & Ashley, L. *Only connect.* Toronto: Oxford University Press, 1969.

Eliot, T. S. *The sacred wood.* London: Methuen & Co., 1976.

Farmer, P. Jorinda and Jorindel and other stories. *Children's literature in education.* 1972, *7,* 10–14.

Ferguson, C., & Slobin, D. (Eds.). *Studies of child language development.* New York: Holt, Rinehart & Winston, 1973.

Fernald, C. D. Control of grammar in imitation, comprehension, and production: Problems of replication. *Journal of Verbal Learning & Verbal Behavior,* 1972, *11,* 606–613.

Fillmore, C. J. The case for case. In E. Bach & R. T. Harms (Eds.), *Universals in linguistic theory.* New York: Holt, Rinehart & Winston, 1968.

Fodor, J., & Garrett, M. Some syntactic determinants of sentential complexity. *Perception and psychophysics,* 1967, *2,* 289–296.

Fodor, J., & Katz, J. (Eds.). *The structure of language: Readings in the philosophy of language.* Englewood Cliffs, NJ: Prentice Hall, 1965.

Foster, R., Giddan, J., & Stark, J. *Assessment of child's language comprehension.* Palo Alto: Consulting Psychologists Press, 1973.

Fraser, C., Bellugi, U., & Brown, R. Control of grammar in imitation, comprehension and production. In R. C. Oldfield & J. C. Marshall (Eds.), *Language.* Baltimore: Penguin Books, 1968.

Fries, C. C. *Linguistics and reading.* New York: Holt, Rinehart & Winston, 1966.

Frye, N. *On teaching literature.* New York: Harcourt, Brace, Jovanovich, 1972.

Furth, H. *Thinking without language: Psychological implications of deafness.* New York: Free Press, 1966.

Furth, H. Linguistic deficiency and thinking: Research with deaf subjects, 1964–1969. *Psychological Bulletin,* 1971, *76,* 58–72.

Furth, H. *Deafness and learning: A social-developmental psychology.* Belmont, CA: Wadsworth, 1972.

Gans, R. *Guiding children's reading through experience.* New York: Teachers College Press, 1963.

Gibson, E., & Levin, H. *The psychology of reading.* Cambridge, MA: M.I.T. Press, 1975.

Gibson, E., Shurcliff, A., & Yonas, A. Utilization of spelling patterns by deaf and hearing subjects. In H. Levin & J. Williams (Eds.), *Basic studies in reading.* New York: Basic Books, 1970.

Goodman, K. S. Reading: A psycholinguistic guessing game. *Journal of the Reading Specialist,* 1967, *4,* 126–135.

Grégoire, A. *L'Apprentissage du langage: Les deux premières années.* Paris: Librairie E. Droz, 1937.

Guilford, J. Frontiers in thinking. *The Reading Teacher,* 1960, *13,* 229–231.

Gundlach, R., & Moses, R. *Developmental issues in the study of children's written language.* Paper presented at the First Annual Boston University Conference on Language Development, 1976.

Guszak, F. Teacher questioning and reading. *The Reading Teacher,* 1967, *21,* 12–19.

Harris, Z. S. *Methods in structural linguistics.* Chicago: University of Chicago Press, 1951.

Harris, Z. S. Co-occurrence and transformation in linguistic structure. In J. Fodor & J. Katz (Eds.), *The structure of language: Readings in the philosophy of language.* Englewood Cliffs, NJ: Prentice Hall, 1965.

Hart, B. O. *Teaching reading to deaf children.* Washington, D.C.: A. G. Bell Assoc. 1963.

Herber, H. *Teaching reading in content areas.* Englewood Cliffs, NJ: Prentice Hall, 1970.

Huttenlocher, J. K., & Strauss, S. Comprehension: Relation between perceived actor & logical subject. *Journal of Verbal Learning & Verbal Behavior,* 1968, *7,* 300–304.

Jacobs, R., & Rosenbaum, P. *English transformational grammar.* Waltham, MA: Blaisdell (Ginn), 1968.

Jacobs, R., & Rosenbaum, P. S. (Eds.). *Transformations, style and meaning.* Waltham, MA: Xerox College Publishing, 1971.

Jacobovits, L., & Miron, M. (Eds.). *Readings in the psychology of language.* Englewood Cliffs, NJ: Prentice Hall, 1967.

Jakobson, R. *Child language, aphasia and phonological universals.* The Hague: Mouton, 1968.

Jakobson, R. Linguistics and poetics. In T. Sebeok (Ed.), *Style in language.* Cambridge, MA: M.I.T. Press, 1969.

Janson, H. W. *History of art for young people.* New York: Abrams, 1971.

Kavanaugh, J., & Cutting, J. E. (Eds.). *The role of speech in language.* Cambridge, MA: M.I.T. Press, 1975.

Kavanaugh, J., & Mattingly, I. (Eds.). *Language by ear and by eye.* Cambridge, MA: M.I.T. Press, 1972.

Kemp, J., & Dale, P. *Spontaneous imitation and free speech: A grammatical comparison.* Paper presented to the Society for Research in Child Development, Philadelphia, March, 1973.

Koch, K. *Wishes, lies and dreams.* New York: Chelsea House, 1970.

Koch, K. *Rose, where did you get that red?* New York: Vintage Books, 1973.

Kohl, H. *Reading, how to.* New York: Bantam Books, 1973.

Lee, L., & Canter, S. M. Developmental sentence scoring. *Journal of Speech and Hearing Disorders,* 1971, *36,* 315–338.

Lenneberg, E. Understanding language without ability to speak: A case report. *Journal of Abnormal and Social Psychology,* 1962, *65,* 419–425.

Leopold, W. *Speech development of a bilingual child: A linguist's record. Grammar and general problems in the first two years.* Vol. III Evanston, IL: Northwestern University Press, 1949.

Lopate, P. *On being with children.* New York: Dell, 1976.

Lovell, K., & Dixon, E. The growth of the control of grammar in imitation, comprehension, and production. *Journal of Child Psychology & Psychiatry,* 1967, *8,* 31–39.

Man: A course of study. Washington, DC: Curriculum Development Associates, 1966.

McCarthy, D. Language development in children. In L. Carmichael (Ed.), *Manual of child psychology.* New York: Wiley & Sons, 1954.

McElhanon, K. A. (Ed.). *Legends from Papua New Guinea.* Ukarumpa: Summer Institute of Linguistics, 1974.

McNeill, D. Developmental psycholinguistics. In F. Smith & G. Miller (Eds.), *The genesis of language: A psycholinguistic approach.* Cambridge, MA: M.I.T. Press, 1966.

McNeill, D. *The acquisition of language: The study of developmental psycholinguistics.* New York: Harper & Row, 1970.

Menyuk, P. Syntactic rules used by children from pre-school through first-grade. *Child development,* 1964, *35,* 533–546.

Menyuk, P. *Sentences children use.* Cambridge, MA: M.I.T. Press, 1969.

Menyuk, P. *The acquisition and development of language.* Englewood Cliffs, NJ: Prentice Hall, 1971.

Miller, G. A. Some preliminaries to psycholinguistics (1965). In L. Jakobovits, & M. Miron (Eds.), *Readings in the psychology of language.* Englewood Cliffs, NJ: Prentice Hall, 1967.

Milne, A. A. *The house at Pooh corner.* New York: E. P. Dutton, 1961.

Moffett, J. *A student-centered language arts curriculum, grades K-6: A handbook for teachers.* Boston: Houghton-Mifflin, 1973.

Moore, T. E. (Ed.). *Cognitive development and the acquisition of language.* New York: Academic Press, 1973.

Nelson, K. Structure and strategy in learning to talk. *Monographs of the Society for Research in Child Development,* 1973, *38,* No. 149.

Newsome, V. *Structural grammar in the classroom.* Champlain, IL: National Council of Teachers of English, 1967.

Oléron, P. Recherches sur le development mental des sourdsmuets. *Centre National de la Recherche Scientifique,* Paris, 1957.

Oléron, P. Conceptual thinking of the deaf. In P. Adams (Ed.), *Language in thinking.* Baltimore: Penguin Books, Ltd., 1972.

Osgood, C. E. Motivational dynamics of language behavior. In M. R. Jones (Ed.), *Nebraska Symposium on Motivation.* Lincoln: University of Nebraska Press, 1957.

Paraskevopoulous, K., & Kirk, S. *The development and psychometric characteristics of the revised Illinois Test of Psycholinguistic Abilities.* Urbana: University of Illinois Press, 1969.

Parker, E. A. *Teaching the reading of fiction.* New York: Teachers College Press, 1969.

Piaget, J. *The construction of reality in the child.* New York: Basic Books, 1954 (1st Edition, 1926).

Piaget, J. *Judgment and reasoning in the child.* New York: Littlefield, Adams, & Co., 1928.

Piaget, J. *The origins of intelligence in children.* New York: International Universities Press, 1952 (1st Edition, 1936).

Piaget, J. *The language and thought of the child.* New York: Meridian Books, 1955.

Piaget, J. *The origins of intelligence in children.* New York: Norton & Co., Inc., 1963.

Piaget, J. *The child's conception of number.* New York: Norton & Co., Inc., 1965.

Quigley, S., & Power, D. Deaf children's acquisition of passive voice. *Journal of Speech and Hearing Research,* 1973, *16,* 5–11.

Quigley, S., Russell, K., & Power, D. *Linguistics and deaf children: Transformational syntax and its application.* Washington, D.C.: A.G. Bell Assoc., 1976.

Report, Rhode Island School for the Deaf, 1879–1900.

Roberts, P. *English syntax.* New York: Harcourt, Brace, & World, 1964.

Roberts, P. *The Roberts English series: A linguistic program for grades 3–8.* New York: Harcourt, Brace & World, Inc., 1966.

Roche Report: *Frontiers of hospital psychiatry,* Oct. 1, 1967.

Rosenbaum, P. *The grammar of English predicate complement constructions.* Cambridge, MA: M.I.T. Press, 1967.

Rosenheim, E. W. Children's reading & adults' values. In S. Egoff (Ed.), *Only connect.* Toronto: Oxford University Press, 1969.

Ross, J. R. *Constraints on variables in syntax.* Unpublished doctoral dissertation, M.I.T. Department of Linguistics, 1967.

Ross, J. R. On declarative sentences. In R. Jacobs, & P. Rosenbaum (Eds.), *Readings in English transformational grammar.* Waltham: Blaisdell Press, 1970.

Ross, J. R. Parallels in phonological and semantic organization. In J. F. Kavanaugh, & J. E. Cutting (Eds.), *The role of speech in language.* Cambridge, MA: M.I.T. Press, 1975.

Samuels, S. J. Modes of word recognition. In H. Singer & R. Ruddell (Eds.), *Theoretical models and processes in reading.* Newark: International Reading Association, 1970.

Schlesinger, I. M. Production of utterances and language acquisition. In D. I. Slobin (Ed.), *The ontogenesis of grammar: A theoretical symposium.* New York: Academic Press, 1971.

Scholes, R. *Structuralism in literature.* New Haven: Yale University Press, 1974.

Sigel, I. E., Anderson, L., & Shapiro, H. Categorization behavior of lower and middle-class Negro pre-school children: Differences in dealing with representation of familiar objects. *Journal of Negro Education,* 1966, *35,* 129–150.

Silverman, T. Unpublished paper presented at the *Conference of Executives of American Schools for the Deaf.* Washington, D.C., 1968.

Sinclair-de-Zwart, H. Developmental psycholinguistics. In D. Elkind, & J. Flavell (Eds.), *Studies in cognitive development.* New York: Oxford University Press, 1969.

Sinclair-de-Zwart, H. Language acquisition and cognitive development. In T. E. Moore (Ed.), *Cognitive development and the acquisition of language.* New York: Academic Press, 1973.

Sloan, G. D. *The child as critic.* New York: Teachers College Press, 1975.

Slobin, D. I. Developmental psycholinguistics. In W. O. Dingwall (Ed.), *A survey of linguistic science.* College Park: University of Maryland Press, 1971.

Slobin, D. I. Cognitive prerequisites for the development of grammar. In C. Ferguson & D. Slobin (Eds.), *Studies of child language development.* New York: Holt, Rinehart & Winston, 1973.

Slobin, D. I., & Welsh, C. Elicited imitations as a research tool in developmental psycholinguistics. In C. A. Ferguson & D. Slobin (Eds.), *Studies of child language development.* New York: Holt, Rinehart & Winston, 1973.

Smith, F. *Psycholinguistics and reading.* New York: Holt, Rinehart & Winston, 1970.

Smith, F. The role of prediction in reading. *Elementary English.* 1975, *52,* 305–311.

Stokoe, W. C., Jr. The shape of soundless language. In J. Kavanaugh & J. Cutting (Eds.), *The role of speech in language.* Cambridge, MA: M.I.T. Press, 1975.

Stokoe, W. C., Jr. Sign language structure. *Studies in linguistics.* Occasional Papers No. 8. Buffalo: Buffalo University Press, 1960.

Vygotsky, L. S. *Thought and language.* Cambridge, MA: M.I.T. Press, 1962 (1st Edition, 1934).

Weiner, M., & Cromer, J. Reading difficulty: A conceptual analysis. *Harvard Educational Review,* 1967, *34,* 620–637.

BIBLIOGRAPHY OF CHILDREN'S LITERATURE

Blume, J. *Tales of a fourth grade nothing.* New York: Dell, 1972.

Craig, M. J. *The three wishes.* New York: Scholastic Book Services, 1968.

D'Aulaire, M. *Trolls.* New York: Doubleday & Co., 1972.

George, J. *My side of the mountain.* New York: E. P. Dutton, 1959.

Grahame, K. *The wind in the willows.* New York: Dell Books, 1969.

Heins, P. (Translator). *Snow White by the Brothers Grimm.* Boston: Atlantic Monthly Press, 1974.

Juster, N. *The phantom tollbooth.* New York: Random House, 1961.

Kennedy, R. *Come again in the spring.* New York: Harper & Row, 1976.

Konigsberg, E. L. *Jennifer, Hecate, Macbeth, William McKinley and me, Elizabeth.* New York: Atheneum, 1967.

Lippman, P. *The great escape.* New York: Golden Press, 1973.

Mann, P. *My dad lives in a downtown hotel.* New York: Camelot Books, 1973.

Mayer, M. *A special trick.* New York: Dial Press, 1970.

McDermott, G. *Arrow to the sun.* New York: Penguin Books, 1977.

McGovern, A. *Stone soup.* New York: Scholastic Book Services, 1968.

Sendak, M. *Where the wild things are.* New York: Harper & Row, 1963.

Shapiro, I. *The golden book of the Renaissance.* New York: Golden Press, 1961.

Shulevitz, U. *One monday morning,* New York: Scribner & Sons, 1967.

Silverstein, S. *The giving tree.* New York: Harper & Row, 1964.

Steiner, J., & Mueller, J. *The bear who wanted to be a bear.* New York: Atheneum, 1976.

Ungerer, T. *The three robbers.* New York: Atheneum Press, 1962.

White, E. B. *Charlotte's web.* New York: Harper & Row, 1952.

Wilde, O. *The selfish giant.* London: Spring Books, 1963.

Zindel, P. *The pigman,* New York: Dell, 1968.

INDEX

M

N

O

P

Q

R

S

T

V

W